The Natural Beauty Book
Cruelty-free cosmetics to make at home

The Natural Beauty Book

Anita Guyton

Thorsons
An Imprint of HarperCollins*Publishers*

Thorsons
An Imprint of HarperCollins*Publishers*
77-85 Fulham Palace Road,
Hammersmith, London W6 8JB

First published by Thorsons 1981 as
The Book of Natural Beauty
Revised, expanded and redesigned edition published
1984 as *The Woman's Book of Natural Beauty*
This revised and redesigned edition published 1991
10 9 8 7 6 5

Illustrations by Denise Scourfield

A catalogue record for this book
is available from the British Library

ISBN 0 7225 2498 6

Typeset by Harper Phototypesetters Limited
Northampton, England
Printed in Great Britain by
Woolnough Bookbinding Limited,
Irthlingborough, Northamptonshire

To a very beautiful woman — my mother.

Contents

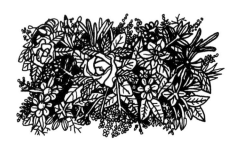

Introduction

For well over 5,000 years women have pampered and adorned themselves in the belief that they may attain the 'ideal combination of qualities which delight the sight' — otherwise referred to as beauty. Today, this quest is still relentlessly pursued.

Throughout history, famous beauties have used natural cosmetics, yet many sceptics still argue that the aids they employed failed to prevent their features from ageing. This argument is partly true, but no cosmetics, however effective, could stem the harmful effects of insanitary living conditions, infrequent bathing, unhealthy diets and poorly ventilated homes, all of which were prevalent and which helped to produce a breeding ground for germs. These environmental and personal factors frequently resulted in debilitating and deadly diseases, one of them being smallpox, which invariably left bad scars.

Some cosmetics were extracted from plants and animal products, but others — such as the lead-based white powders and pastes fashionable in Elizabethan times — were not only impure but dangerous. When used frequently they actually harmed the complexion and severely damaged health.

During the greater part of the twentieth century, marketing men have tried to tempt and entice us into purchasing elaborately packed and consequently expensive creams and lotions with the promise that these mass-manufactured chemical potions will turn our dreams of physical perfection into reality. To maintain and increase sales they regularly resort to attacking home-made preparations, but many women have become disillusioned with commercial products and are turning to herbs, spices, fruit, vegetables and other natural ingredients, in the hope that the resulting preparations will prove less harmful, less expensive and more beneficial than their largely synthetic counterparts. One reason why I use only nature's products has to do with the growing concern at animal exploitation in the beauty industry, from the inclusion of fats such as whale oil in cosmetics to the frequent use made of harmless little creatures in painful laboratory experiments — but this is not the only reason. There is no short cut to beauty, but from my own experiments and personal experiences I am convinced there is only one sure step towards it. That is to incorporate such ingredients as honey, almonds, cream, egg, yogurt and vegetable oils into our daily beauty routine.

My reason for writing this book is to encourage and help those interested in this ancient, yet relatively undiscovered, world of beauty, for I believe most women would look more attractive, many quite lovely, and some beautiful if they pursued and applied these daily home beauty treatments. This practice could undoubtedly have a far-reaching and positive effect on their lives, leading to a greater self-awareness. A well-groomed woman who not only thinks and feels, but knows she looks attractive is consequently more confident, and this inner sureness and outer glow frequently leads to greater security and a happier and fuller life.

These cosmetics and toiletries (many of which are my own recipes, whilst others have been in my family for generations) are fun and inexpensive to make and absolutely delicious to use. But, most importantly, they give excellent results.

PART ONE

Ingredients

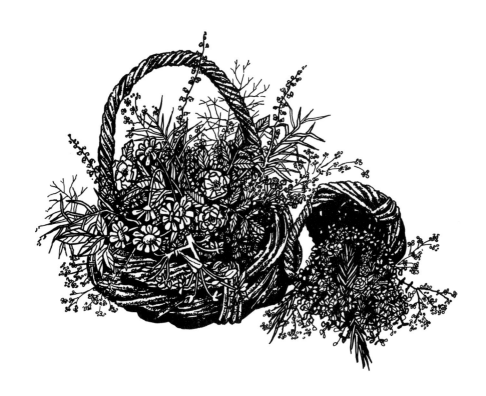

1
Container Growing

When growing herbs, plants, or shrubs in containers, it is wise to consider the physical limitations of your home before choosing the holders. Flat dwellers with a small balcony will generally be well advised to install some 'ledge' boxes, a few hanging baskets, which take up no precious floor space, and the odd tub or two. Living in a flat without a balcony or verandah limits one to indoor and outdoor window boxes, and hanging baskets. Together these can provide a fair supply of fresh herbs and small plants. Some houses and cottages, particularly those in country districts, will have a fair-sized garden in which a particular border can be devoted entirely to varieties destined to be used for your new, natural beauty programme. And town houses with small patio-type yards can supply a regular herbal harvest — and look extremely charming and colourful — with a selection of window boxes, hanging baskets, strawberry barrels and other tubs of different designs, shapes, and sizes.

Holders originally designed for mundane domestic uses, such as sinks, tin baths, wash basins and the like, can be brightened up and made to look attractive.

Container growing is indeed an art, combining man-made effort with natural foliage and flowers. In the beginning it is very much like attempting to powder, paint and so transform a so-called 'plain' woman into a beautiful one, for the container, like skin, has to be sound, clean and prepared.

All containers should have good drainage. The excess moisture that builds up in a watertight holder will cause plants to rot, and the compost will quickly become stale and sour. Approximately twelve good-sized holes to every square foot of floor area will suffice, and these should be drilled and distributed evenly along the container floor.

Unless your containers are made of plastic or nylon, your next thought must be to protect and preserve them, both inside and out, against the damaging effects of day-to-day watering and exposure to the elements. In the past, the insides of wooden troughs were preserved in the traditional way: by charring them. Nothing seems to last quite so long as partially burned wood, and a blowlamp will do the job efficiently in minutes. If there's no such tool available, take the container into either an open part of the garden well away from your neighbours' or on to a patch of wasteland where there is nothing inflammable nearby. Pack the inside of the trough lightly with a few sheets of dried newspaper and then light it. When the inside is evenly charred and browned, tip the container upside down with a long-handled tool, and the flames will quickly be extinguished. Using a wood preservative is a safe and very much cleaner method, but make sure that you use a horticulturally approved brand, thus ensuring that it will not harm your plants. Creosote should never be used. Tin or metal holders are best treated inside and out first with an undercoat of paint and then with two top coats. Plain metal hanging baskets will look better and last much longer if given the same treatment, but those protected by a plastic covering will need no 'doctoring'.

Many containers, such as concrete tubs, apart from their lack of drainage holes, are well-suited to growing house plants. This lack of porosity can be partially remedied by 'crocking' the inside of the container with a quantity of broken brick, stones and gravel, up to at least one-quarter of its inside depth. Tall barrels and tubs in which only small plants are to be grown can obviously take a far greater proportion without any likelihood of the plants suffering root starvation. Boxes with drainage holes must also be provided with a layer of clean crocks, and when using tubs, boxes and similar containers, always add some charcoal granules to keep the compost sweet.

There are several different compost mixtures in which herbs and small plants grow very well, though all have some qualities in common. Evenly blended compost must be sterilized and nutritious, yet light and porous. This enables the roots to breathe and feed whilst allowing excess moisture to drain away freely.

Herbs and small plants do well in such mixtures as: two parts of JIP (John Innes Potting compost) No. 2, two parts of peat and one part of well-rotted leafmould; *or* three parts of JIP No. 3, two parts of peat and two parts of coarse sand; *or* two parts of JIP No. 2, two parts of peat, one part of coarse sand and one part of well-rotted leafmould. Larger shrubs and small trees always benefit from a somewhat richer mixture, such as three parts of JIP No. 3, two parts of rotted leafmould, one part of peat and one part of coarse sand.

In rural areas, cut turves are far more readily available than in towns. Even if you are only able to acquire a few rough ones to line your window boxes and barrels, it will be well worth the trouble. As they slowly rot, they provide a wonderfully rich source of food for growing plants. Turves should be placed evenly on top of the crocks, grass side facing downwards, before filling the containers to within an inch or two of the top with your chosen compost. You should first line hanging baskets with either sphagnum moss (available from florists and gardening centres) or turves, which in this case should be set so that the grass side is facing inwards. Then add a little JIP No. 2 or 3 compost, before arranging and setting your plants firmly into place using more compost. To allow sufficient space for watering, the growing medium should only reach to within a half to one inch (1.5–3 cm) of the brim of the pot.

Marigolds and many of the tinier herbs grow very well together in hanging baskets, but in the warm places they like best they can quickly dry and become parched. To ensure that they remain green and healthy, they should be lifted down and left to soak in a bucket of tepid water for an hour or two each evening before being hoisted back into the warm summer air. All-over spraying will also help to keep them fresh and moist. This should be done early in the morning, before the sun is high in the sky.

To obtain plant displays that both look attractive and provide a good harvest of petals and foliage for cosmetic purposes, it is doubly important to ensure that you get the very best from any mixed planting arrangement. You would be well advised first to categorize your plants into two distinct types, the sun-lovers and those which prefer to grow in partial shade. Then keep the types to themselves, sun-lovers in one container and shade-lovers in another. Only in this way can each be provided with near-perfect growing conditions.

Remember the importance of securely fastening those containers that will either be sitting outside on high window ledges, or hanging well above floor level. Although they may appear quite steady on windless days, it is surprising how unstable they become when storms and high winds are blowing. Once crocked and filled with compost they are heavy, and if they should fall from any great height, you can imagine their dangerous force at the point of impact! Some unfortunate person passing below could all too easily be seriously injured. So always make sure that containers are securely double-fastened with either wedges and hooks or chains and brackets.

Growing herbs indoors
Those who have had success with houseplants are generally far better suited to cultivating herbs indoors, for the basic principles concerning lighting, watering, humidity, temperature and draughts apply equally to both. Like houseplants, herbs can be grown indoors in hanging baskets, pots, tubs and troughs, but the position that you allot them must be right. Light, for instance, is essential if any plant is to grow, but light that we may consider ideal is often insufficient for plants. Even clean glass windows reduce the amount of natural light entering a room, and the light may be further diminished by net curtaining. Plants also suffer in rooms that reflect little light, either because of a lack of large mirrors, or a dark decor.

It is relatively simple to water plants out of doors but immediately they are contained in pots and brought inside the problem of overwatering may arise. Despite all the books on houseplant care, overwatering is one of the principal reasons for the early demise of plants, but by keeping two simple rules the problem can be eliminated. The most important is to pour water only into the drip tray underneath the container, and then only when the compost looks and feels dry. Secondly, plants must never be allowed to sit in a drip tray full of water for more than one and a half hours after watering, for this will quickly cause the roots to rot.

Indoor-grown herbs, like houseplants, need a humid atmosphere in which to thrive, and although maintaining this may at first seem difficult, the solution is really quite easy. Successful indoor gardeners use one of a number of simple techniques. Buying a humidifier for each room is one solution. Another is to stand the potted herbs on a deepish watertight tray, the base of which is first covered with an inch or so of clean pebbles. Next, pour on barely enough water to cover the floor of the container, without it reaching either the top of the stones or the base of the pots; otherwise the plants' confined roots will quickly become waterlogged, rot and die. Individual specimens whose plain pots are hidden by more attractive outer holders may be treated by packing the gap between the plain pot and the decorative container with wet sphagnum moss or peat. By regularly topping up the water level in the tray, or moistening the moss between the walls of the pots, the herbs will be assured of a constantly rising damp atmosphere. This will prevent them turning brown (often referred to as 'dry air damage') and keep them in peak condition.

When it comes to temperature, try to steer a middle course for, as with most growing things, herbs dislike fluctuations in room temperature. I have found it unwise to keep them in the living room, or indeed in any room that is used every day, because a temperature that we humans consider comfortable and cosy (around 75°F/24°C) is far too warm for herbs. There is little sense in our feeling miserably chilly just because the plants prefer it that way, so the best alternative is to confine indoor gardening to a spare room where the temperature remains fairly static at between 55°F and 65°F (12°C and 18°C). Thus you can avoid the sudden rises and falls in temperature that frequently prove fatal to all types of plants.

If, like me, you both work and sleep with at least one window open, summer and winter, your 'cosmetics-to-be greenery' will not suffer from lack of fresh air. A constant flow of clean, pure air is always necessary. Draughts, however, are a different matter. When plants are positioned directly in front of either a constantly opening door or a badly fitting window, both of which permit passage of cold air, the results are 'chilling' and the herbs quickly sicken and often die.

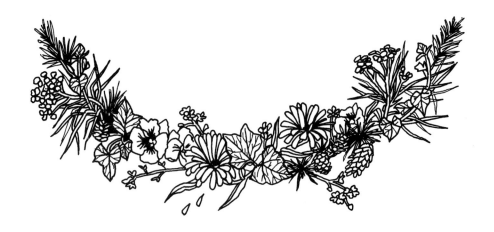

2
Harvesting, Drying and Storage

There is something thrilling about harvesting all the fresh natural produce that you intend to use in cosmetics and toiletries. The excitement and satisfaction is like that of a chef or someone who goes into the garden to select and gather herbs and vegetables rather than opening packets or tins of processed foods. This simile does not finish there, because just as the body must be internally nourished with a variety of fresh foods to ensure general good health, so your skin needs various forms of external nourishment to stay young and vital.

Whether the herbs or plants are to be picked from your own garden or from the wild, only harvest those flowers, leaves and roots that are fresh and in peak condition — the sprigs of herbs should be young, the blossoms freshly opened, the leaves newly unfurled and the roots gathered only in mid-autumn or early spring, when they contain all the food reserves necessary for new growth.

It is worth choosing your day for harvesting carefully, the best time being early on a dry morning, when enough warmth has dispelled the night dew but not yet started to dry the valuable oils contained in the top growth. Always avoid gathering polluted plants growing alongside main roads, only pick sufficient for your needs and never handle them any more than is absolutely necessary. Go armed, preferably with a gardener's trug, a flat-bottomed basket, or a clean tray or two, and having gathered your sprigs, sprays and blossoms lay them flat. This is much more important than you think, because only by treating them gently to prevent bruising and crushing can you be sure of retaining their much-prized and beautifying oils and juices. Polythene bags, being light, perhaps seem a practical means of collecting, but as well as allowing the fruits of your labours to be easily damaged, the man-made polythene imprisons heat, which causes the produce to wilt and decompose within hours.

17

Drying herbs

Never strip the aromatic leaves from the herbs you have picked, but place the whole sprays in light hessian or net curtaining, or lay them carefully on airy slatted trays that have linings of nylon or stainless steel gauze.

Having prepared your herbs, the drying process itself must be completed as quickly as possible, and in the dark, thus retaining all their perfume and oils. The most practical way of achieving this is to place the herbs either in an airing cupboard or a warm oven, where the temperature must not exceed 90°F (32°C). Hotter than this, they could become discoloured and lose their flavour. Each tray or cloth should be labelled with the name of the herb, and putting only one herb in every holder will prevent the intermingling of aromas and plants. Once dry, they are not always easily recognizable.

During the drying itself, the first twenty-four hours are the most vital. The herbs should be turned several times to ensure that they are drying evenly. Once dry — that is when they feel crisp and break whenever handled — they should be removed from the oven or cupboard, rubbed together with cotton-gloved hands (the gloves will prevent your hands from becoming chafed) and finally sieved and stored.

Drying flowers and leaves

Flowers and leaves can be treated in the same way, except that flowers need to be handled much more gently. Alternatively, several sprays at a time may be bound together and hung upside down to dry in an attic or other darkened room where there is a free flow of warm air. When dry, petals look entirely free of moisture and rather 'papery' whilst the leaves appear very parched and snap easily. All flowers and petals are stored whole. The leaves, too, may be kept in this way, or may be treated like herbs, first being rubbed between gloved palms and then sieved and potted in airtight storage jars.

Drying roots

Newly lifted roots are first trimmed of all fibrous appendages. They are then sprayed or, if needs be, scrubbed with clean water and left to dry off for an hour or two in a warm room. Next they should be cut into half-inch lengths and placed on slatted trays in a heated oven, the temperature of which should be pre-set at 175°F (80°C, Gas Mark 2). The door should be slightly ajar. When the roots are thoroughly dried, they will be fairly brittle right through and ready to snap at the slightest pressure.

Storing

Herbs keep quite well in either small, home-made hessian-type bags with draw-string cords, or in sealed brown paper bags. Both plants and herbs can be stored in opaque glass storage jars with tight fitting lids. If only clear glass containers are available, ensure that they are stored in a dark and dry place such as the airing cupboard or under a bed. All dried materials will lose much of their natural colour and fragrance if exposed to bright light. Label all containers carefully.

Under no circumstances should tins be employed as containers, for they can often affect the herbs' true flavours. If after a week or more your dried materials collect beads of moisture, the contents of the container must be poured on to a sheet of clean paper immediately and left in a warm, dark room to dry off. Before re-packing remove all condensation from the jar with a warm, dry cloth.

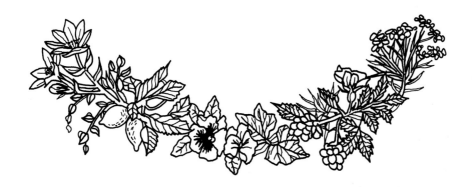

3

Essential and Aromatic Oils

The second part of this book gives instructions for making a wide range of skin and hand creams, hair conditioners, shampoos, and unusual and delightful toiletries, but only where it is essential to the recipe have I included a specific perfumed oil. My reasons for excluding such perfumes from these recipes are twofold. First, many readers might be deterred on discovering that a particular aromatic oil is either too expensive or difficult to obtain. Second, choosing perfumes is a very personal thing: some people adore the smell of one scent whilst others find it less than agreeable.

These were the only reasons for not allocating specific aromas to the recipes, but I fully realize that all these gorgeous bottled lotions and potted concoctions are certainly enhanced by the inclusion of a favourite and subtle-smelling oil. Choose your own and add a few drops before bottling. All sorts of exciting and sensual aromatic oils are obtainable from companies specializing in the production of 'essential' oils.

There is much excitement and fun in making your own cosmetics and toiletries using oils you have bought, and a great deal more if you take the process one step further and produce your own perfumed oils. The end results may not always prove as potent or heady as the commercially marketed ones, but you'll be pleasantly surprised to find how strong they can be, especially once you have gained a little experience and become more adventurous. The oils produced at home will prove extremely good, are considerably less expensive than factory kinds, and another of the many nice things about them is that they can be used lavishly without any fear of breaking the bank!

Herbal oils
First pound your chosen herbs with a crushing tool such as a pestle or grinder, until they are bruised and ground to a coarse powder. Then spoon four tablespoons of these herbs into a clean,

pint-sized (570 ml) jar, add two tablespoons of wine vinegar or vodka, and then pour in sufficient sunflower, almond, or corn oil to fill the jar to within three-quarters of the top.

Screw the lid down tightly, and place it in a warm sunny spot — I line up most of mine on a shelf in the kitchen, not just because the conditions are perfect but also because whenever I go there to prepare a meal I see them displayed so prominently that I am reminded to give them all a good shake! Another ideal place to line a few bottles is immediately above a radiator, for warmth is needed to bring out the natural aroma of the herbs.

After about three weeks, strain the oil, squeeze out the herbs and keep them on one side, for although much of their perfume will have been absorbed by the oil, they usually still have a little scent and oil, which is well worth using in your bath. Now add four more tablespoons of freshly pounded herbs to the strained oil, cork the jar and leave for a further three weeks. Strain the oil again and add some more herbs. Repeat the process until the oil smells as strong and herby as you want.

Finally, pass the oil through a piece of fine gauze or nylon stocking. Bottle and cork it, then label and store it in a dark place. I keep a bottle of herbal oil solely as a bath additive and body oil. After a bath I pour some into the palm of my hand and give myself an all-over massage. It is easily absorbed into the skin, keeping it beautifully supple and silky.

If you intend to build up a good stock of oils — and a wonderfully varied range of smells can be built up over a period of a year or so — do remember always to label each jar immediately you immerse the herbs or indeed any other ingredients, for it is so easy to forget which preparations are which.

Floral oils

Just a fraction more care is necessary in extracting and capturing flower fragrances, but it won't take long and any woman, however busy, should be able to find time to indulge herself and prepare a lovely floral perfume. Really highly scented flowers, such as strains of rose, jasmine, lilac, stocks, and lily of the valley, may be plucked from the garden and wrapped — not crushed — in an airtight polythene bag. These blooms should be used over a period of anything from several hours to two or even three days and the fresher they remain, the better.

To extract the oils, a double boiler is ideal, but if you don't have one you can easily improvise by standing a small heat-resistant pan inside a larger saucepan, with enough water to prevent the contents of the inner chamber being burned. Pour half a pint (285 ml) of either sunflower or sweet almond oil into the smaller pan, and heat the bottom pan until the oil is just nicely warm. Then pack onto the oil sufficient blooms to fill the inner pot, place a tight-fitting lid on it and leave it on an extremely low heat to warm it through gently, no more!

Two hours later, squeeze all the oil from the flowers, remove and replace them with a fresh supply, once again packing them in until the inner container is full. Repeat the process every two hours, until the perfumed oil is of just the right strength. Only then bring the oil and all the blooms to the boil, reduce the heat immediately and allow the oil to simmer until the flowers look crisp and dried up. Finally, squeeze all the oil from the flowers and strain it through fine gauze or nylon. Add one teaspoon of liquid storax and one teaspoon tincture of benzoin. Bottle, cork tightly, shake well, label and store in a dark cupboard.

Tinctures

The resinous substances contained in certain herbs cannot be dissolved and captured by the usual means of either decocting (boiling) or infusing the herbs (as in the making of tea). The only alternative, therefore, is to activate these gum-like 'juices' by soaking the herbs in alcohol, so producing a tincture.

To achieve this, pour sixteen tablespoons of pounded herbs into a large screw-top jar, together with two pints (1.15 litres) of either wine vinegar, surgical spirit or alcohol. Screw down the lid fairly tightly and stand the container in a warm, preferably sunny place, for two weeks. As with essential oils, tinctures need shaking regularly several times a day. After fourteen days, filter, bottle, label and store in a dark cupboard.

Essences

Essences are solely for external application and are made by mixing two tablespoons of an essential oil with one pint (570ml) of either alcohol, wine vinegar or surgical spirit.

Aromatic Oils

Angelica Oil

This pale brown, often almost colourless oil has a strong, peppery, aromatic odour which resembles musk. It is used in perfumes, and is distilled from the roots and/or seeds of the *Archangelica officinalis*, a plant indigenous to Asia and Northern Europe.

Backhousia Oil

This oil possesses a sweet fresh-lemon smell, and is used in the manufacture of soaps and perfumes. It is distilled from the leaves of the *Backhousia citriodora* tree, found growing around Brisbane and Gympie in Queensland, Australia.

Bay Oil

Also known as Myrcia oil, because it is obtained from the leaves of the West Indian *Myrcia acris* shrub or tree. Originally yellow in colour, the oil turns brown by oxidation when exposed to the air. It has a pungent, clove-like perfume, and is used in the manufacture of perfumes, soaps, and Bay Rum.

Bergamot Oil

This yellow to greenish, orangey-smelling oil, is incorporated in eau de colognes, toilet waters and perfumes, and is extracted from the fresh peel of the *Citrus bergamia* fruit. This fruiting tree grows only in the Southern provinces of Calabria and Reggio in Italy.

Bergamot Mint Oil

A yellowish oil which smells somewhat like lavender oil, and is obtained from the *Mentha citrata*. The plant, a member of the mint family, grows in Florida.

Boronia Oil

Produced by distilling the blooms and occasionally the leaves of a shrubby tree which belongs to the *Boronia* species, and is indigenous to West and South West Australia. The oil is green in colour, and has a delightful mixed herbal and floral perfume.

Camomile Oil (Roman)

Camomile oil varies in colour from pale blue to bluish-green, and is distilled from the dried blooms of the Roman Camomile (*Anthemis nobilis*), a wild plant which grows in Great Britain and other parts of Europe. Its flowery aroma is used to perfume hair shampoo, whilst the somewhat bitter flavour is added to certain medicines.

Canadian Snake Root Oil

Obtained from the roots of the *Asarum canadense*, native to the USA and Canada. The oil is yellowish in colour, and gives a certain spicy fragrance to eau de colognes which is somewhat reminiscent of mixed ginger and patchouli oils.

Caraway Oil

It is used to flavour and perfume mouthwashes and toilet soaps, and is the pale yellow oil extracted from the seeds of the biennial *Carum carvi*, a herb which is indigenous to Holland but also grows in North Africa, Germany, England, and other parts of Europe.

Cedar Wood Oil

Light yellow in colour, this oil has a lovely woody fragrance. This is understandable, for it is distilled from the wood of the North American *Juniperus virginiana* tree. it is used in various types of perfumes.

Cinnamon Oil (Ceylon)

This is another aromatic and woody-smelling oil. It is distilled from the bark of the *Cinnamomum zeylanicum* tree, which is a native of Ceylon and the East Indies. Of a dark yellow colour, it is added to perfumes and dental toiletries.

Cinnamon Leaf Oil

Slightly lighter in colour, this one is also produced by the distillation of part of the *Cinnamomum zeylanicum* tree, in this case the leaves and the twigs. It has a spicy clove and cinnamon aroma, and is used in the manufacture of perfumes and soaps.

Clove Oil

Also known as Caryophyllus oil, it is distilled from the dried, tight flower buds of the *Eugenia caryophyllata*. The evergreen is a native of the Molucca Islands (Spice Islands), but is also found growing in Tanzania. As the pale yellow oil ages it becomes darker. Its pungent, spicy perfume and its antiseptic qualities make it a favourite ingredient of toothpastes, mouthwashes, and other dental preparations.

Cucumber Oil

Also known as Gourd oil, it is expressed from the fruit and seeds of the cucumber and pumpkin, and has, as one might expect, the characteristic colour and smell of fresh cucumbers.

Cumin Oil

This colourless or pale yellow oil possesses the same odour as the fruit of the *Cuminum cyminum* plant, from which it is distilled. The plant is to be found in India, Malta and North East Africa.

Curcuma Oil

Often referred to as Turmeric, Curcuma oil is saffron yellow in colour, but once added to an alkali solution, it quickly turns a reddish-brown. It is distilled from the root of the *Curcuma longa*, a plant found growing in China and the East Indies.

Cypress Oil

A yellowish oil which smells very much like ambergris. Distilled from the young twigs and foliage of several strains of Cypress trees, it is a product native to West Asia, but the same trees are also found growing in parts of Europe.

Dill Oil

Another pale-yellow oil, this comes from the ripe fruits of the *Peucedanum graveolens*, a herb which grows in Great Britain, Holland and Germany. It is used to perfume soaps and other toiletries, but is also employed as a herbal flavouring agent.

Eucalyptus Oil

The perfume of this oil varies enormously, because it is extracted from the leaves of differing strains of Eucalyptus. Each strain produces a highly individual perfume, from the lemon-scented oil of the *Eucalyptus citriodora*, to the rose-smelling oil of the *E. macarthuri*. These very lovely trees can be seen growing in Australia and Tasmania.

Fennel Oil

The *Foeniculum dulce* and the *F. sativum* are the plants from which Fennel oil is derived, and they are grown in India, Russia, France and some Mediterranean countries. The oil has a subtle aniseed aroma and is used in soaps and perfumes.

Geranium Oil

Also known as 'Oil of Pelargonium' and 'Rose Geranium Oil', it varies in colour from pale yellow to a yellowish-green. It has a musky, rose-like perfume, and is distilled from various types of Pelargoniums, many of which are cultivated in Spain, Italy, Corsica, North Africa and Southern France.

Ginger Oil

This one is a yellowish-oil which has a fairly hot flavour, used both as a flavouring and perfuming oil. It is distilled from the roots of the *Zingibar officinale* plant, which is cultivated throughout China, Japan, India and Africa.

Grapefruit Oil

An amber-coloured, fresh and sweetly perfumed oil, which is obtained by crushing the fresh peel of the *Citrus decumana* fruit. The tree upon which the fruits are borne grows in Florida, and the oil itself is added to perfumes and colognes.

Guaiacwood Oil

Another amber-coloured oil, which has a sweet rose-like fragrance used in perfumes and soaps. It is distilled from the tall-growing *Bulnesia sarmientii* tree found in Argentina.

Hyssop Oil

Distilled from the *Hyssopus officinalis*, a herb found growing in many Mediterranean countries, this oil adds a delightful fragrance to perfumes and eau de colognes, and is also used to flavour medicines and liqueurs.

Jasmine Oil

Jasmine oil is light yellow to reddish-brown in colour, and possesses the distinctive and sweetly exotic fragrances associated with highly perfumed and beautiful Eastern gardens. Obtained from the flowers of the Spanish *Jasminium grandiflora*, it is a delightful part of many soaps and perfumes.

Lavender Oil

The oil varies from being colourless to yellowish-green, and has the familiar sweet fragrance which characterizes many eau de colognes and lavender soaps. It is distilled from the blooms of the *Lavendula vera* and the *L. offiicinalis* plants, which are natives of the Mediterranean, but which are also cultivated in other parts of Europe including Britain and France.

Lavender Spike Oil

In this case we have a mixed lavender and rosemary-type aroma, but unfortunately the oil is not as fragrant as the ordinary 'Lavender oil'. The colourless to pale-yellow or brownish-yellow liquid is obtained from the flowers of the *Lavendula spica*, a plant found in the mountainous regions of France, Spain, Italy and Yugoslavia. It is used to perfume soaps and other bath preparations.

Lemon Peel Oil

This yellow oil possesses the lovely fragrance of fresh lemons, and is expressed from the peel of ripe *Citrus medica* fruits, which are cultivated throughout the Mediterranean regions.

Mandarin Oil

Another Citrus fruit product, this time expressed from the peel of the *Citrus madurensis*. The small trees are found growing in Sicily and Calambria, and the yellow, sweet orange smelling oil is added to a variety of perfumes, colognes, and toiletries.

Monarda Oil

A yellowish oil with a sweet fragrance which suggests a blend of ambergris and lavender. It is distilled from the *Monarda didyma* which is a native of America, like the other species within the same family.

Myrtle Oil

It possesses the same sweet-smelling aroma as the leaves from which it is distilled, and is yellow to greenish-yellow in colour. The flowering *Myrtus communis* bush is a native of the Mediterranean regions.

Orange Peel Oil

As you will know, this oil has the aroma, colour and taste of oranges, and is expressed from the oily, thick-skinned peel of the *Citrus aurantium* fruits. The trees are found growing throughout the Mediterranean, West Indies, California and South West Africa, and the oil is used to both flavour and perfume toiletries, soaps, scents, brilliantines and cosmetics.

Patchouli Oil

Yellowish-brown or light brown in colour, it imparts a strong and penetrating aroma to scents, soaps, and cosmetics. It is distilled from the sun-dried leaves of the herbacious *Pogostemon patchouli*, a perennial found growing in India, South East Asia and the Philippines.

Peppermint Oil

Surely one of the most popular and pleasing of all oils, the Peppermint varies from a clear white to a somewhat yellowish liquid. It possesses the fresh and cool, typical minty flavour, and is distilled from the blooms of different varieties of *Mentha*. Michigan, in the U.S.A, is the world's largest producer of this oil, which is used to flavour and perfume all sorts of dentifrices, mouthwashes, perfumes, soaps and toilet waters.

Pimento Oil

Also known as 'Allspice', this yellow to yellowish-red/brown oil has a refreshing clove-like perfume. It is prepared from the dried unripe berries of the *Pimenta officinalis*, a plant found in Central America and the West Indies. Apart from being an essential ingredient of Bay Rum, Pimento oil is used as a flavouring agent in some toiletries, and as a scent in the manufacture of soaps and perfumes.

Pine Needle Oil

The perfumed oil is reminiscent of pine forests, and is derived from the cones and needles of several varieties of conifers which grow in the Austrian Tyrol, and North East Russia. It acts as a deodorizer and germicide, and imparts a refreshing smell to all types of bath toiletries.

Rose Oil

This oil, also known as 'Otto of Roses', varies in colour from pale yellow to light green and red, and its delightful floral fragrance has made it one of the most sought after for centuries. It is distilled from the red-flowering *Rosa Damascena* shrub, which is found in Morocco, Bulgaria and Anatolia.

Rosewood Oil

Rosewood oil is more frequently referred to as 'Rhodium', and the pure and natural variety is distilled from the wood of the *Convolvulus scoparius*, found in the Canary Islands. Unfortunately, some oils bearing this description are carefully blended mixtures of sandal-wood, palmarosa, and geranium oils.

Sage Oil

This yellow to greenish-yellow oil has a pleasingly warm, herbal type of aroma, and is a flavouring agent as well as being used in the perfumery and soap-making industries. The *Salvia officinalis* herb, from which it is distilled, is native to the northern parts of the Mediterranean.

Sandalwood Oil

'Santal' and 'Sandal' oil are other names for this oil because it is distilled from the roots and inner wood of the *Santalum album*, an evergreen tree which is a native of India and Indonesia. The oil has a haunting, woody aroma, evocative of the East, and is used extensively in the manufacture of soaps and perfumes.

Sassafras Oil

Yellowish in colour, it is used in the perfumery trade, and comes from the roots of the *Sassafras officinale* tree which is native to North America.

Ylang-Ylang Oil

Also know as the 'Cananga Java' oil, this flowery-smelling oil is employed in many of the more expensive perfumes, and is a distillation of the blooms of the *Cananga odorata* tree. The latter is indigenous to the Malay Archipelago, but is cultivated throughout Java and the Philippines.

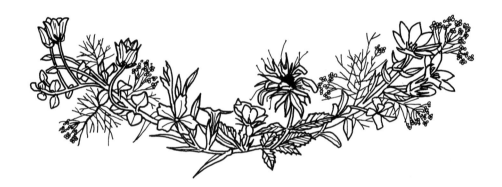

PREPARATIONS USING HERBAL AND FLORAL OILS

Cypress Oil Cream for Varicose Veins

20 teaspoonsful
sweet almond oil
5 teaspoonsful white
wax
¾ teaspoonful
tincture of benzoin
½ teaspoonful
cypress oil

Place the ingredients one at a time in a double boiler or similar container, over a low heat, stirring together gently. When cool, pot up and label. Gently apply the cream to the affected areas.

Juniper Oil for Acne

100 drops olive oil
10 drops juniper
essence

Mix the ingredients together and apply to the affected parts.

Lavender Alcohol for Acne

8 teaspoonsful
alcohol (80 per
cent proof)
½ teaspoonful
lavender essence

Shake the ingredients together thoroughly, before applying to the affected areas. In this and other recipes where alcohol is specified, vodka can be used instead.

Lavender Cream for Acne

50 teaspoonsful
sweet almond oil
13 teaspoonsful
white wax
39 teaspoonsful
distilled water
1 teaspoonful
lavender essence
¼ teaspoonful aspic

Mix the ingredients together slowly, one at a time, in a double boiler or similar container, over a low heat. When cool, pot up and label.

Lavender Oil for the Bath

Put some crushed lavender flowers into a screw-capped jar, and cover completely with almond oil. Stir the contents once a day, always remembering to replace the lid after each stirring. After fourteen days, strain, and bottle. Add a few drops to the bath water.

Lavender flowers
(crushed)
Almond oil

Lemon Essence Cream for Wrinkles

Mix the ingredients together slowly, one at a time, in a double boiler or similar container, over a low heat. When cool, pot up and label.

25 teaspoonsful sweet almond oil
6 teaspoonsful white wax
¾ teaspoonsful tincture of benzoin
19 teaspoonsful distilled water
½ teaspoonsful lemon essence

Lemon Oil for Brittle Nails

Mix the ingredients together. Soak the nails for twenty minutes every evening in the warm lemon oil.

100 drops warm olive oil
10 drops lemon essence

Marigold Oil for Chapped Hands

Put some marigold petals into a screw-capped jar, and cover completely with almond oil. Stir occasionally. Leave for a few days, and then strain and bottle. Pour a little of the marigold oil into the palm of one hand, and work it into the rough and chapped skin.

Marigold petals
Almond oil

4

In the Garden

Angelica (Angelica archangelica)

The origin of this plant's generic name is somewhat uncertain. One theory is that it always flowers on May 8 (the day of Michael the Archangel), whilst another refers to a vision of the Archangel declaring that the plague could be cured by using angelica. The plant is believed to have originated in Syria and it arrived in Britain between 1550 and 1568. It was generally extolled for its medicinal properties and was used by Parkinson, the apothecary of James I, in 1629. When the plague broke out in 1665, the Royal College of Surgeons published a recipe for 'angelica water', which was believed to stave off the fatal sickness.

An extremely robust biennial or perennial, which may reach a height of over nine feet (3 metres), it has become naturalized in most parts of Europe. It has a charming aroma and the greenish-white clusters of flowers appear during the Summer. Packeted seeds for sowing are available from most plant nurseries and garden centres. The dried leaves and roots are sold at herb stockists.

The leaves used in conjunction with other herbal additives make an effective foot-bath, and a sensuously exotic bath mixture. When chewed, the root is effective in eliminating all traces of bad breath.

Bay, sweet bay, Roman laurel, true laurel (Laurus nobilis)

Throughout the ages bay has been considered a protection against evil spirits, as well as a symbol of success. Roman emperors always wore sprigs of bay, especially during violent thunderstorms when they believed that some misfortune might befall them. This belief in its 'divine' power later gave birth to the superstition that when a bay shrub died, a great tragedy was imminent. Bay has long been appreciated for both its culinary and antiseptic properties and has been cultivated in Britain since the sixteenth century.

It is an evergreen shrub with shiny, aromatic, mid-green leathery leaves, which produces clusters of yellowish-green flowers in spring. If left unrestricted in a sunny spot within the shade of some trees, it may reach a height of nearly twenty feet (6 metres). Most horticultural nurseries keep at least two or three standard shrubs on display and, considering that they are somewhat slow-growing, they are usually quite reasonably priced.

Bay leaves can be made up into a variety of exotic bath essences and perfumes, all of which will leave your skin sensuously fragrant and silky soft.

Blackberry *(Rubus fructicosus)*

The blackberry has many popular names such as 'scaldhead', 'bramble', 'bumble', 'brummel', 'brambleberry', and 'bramle-kite', many of which appear to have originated from the Anglo-Saxon word 'bremel' which is possibly a derivative of 'brambel' or 'brymbyl', meaning 'prickly'. The Ancient Greeks were not backward in appreciating this rambler, because as well as eating it purely for pleasure, the fruits were taken to alleviate gout. The blackberry's nickname, 'scaldhead', is particularly applicable, for in times gone by, and even in some country districts today, the leaves are still used as a panacea for all types of burns.

The stems of this tough and woody perennial are usually covered with spines. In early Summer a mass of attractive white flowers are borne on the boughs of the previous year's growth. These blooms are self-fertile, and later give rise to a harvest of round, soft, black fruits.

Plants are available from fruit/plant nurseries and gardening supply centres.

The mass-produced, so called 'natural' cosmetics, rarely contain any part of the blackberry, yet the fruit may be made into a facial which, though a bit squashy, really brings the colour to wan cheeks. Once steeped in water, the leaves quickly provide a multi-purpose beauty aid, either as a mild yet bracing facial astringent, or as a 'pick-me-up' foot or tonic bath. You'll find the bath gel which I have also included is different, and certainly has a way with skin problems!

Carrot *(Daucus carota)*

This root vegetable was quite familiar to the Ancient Greeks and Romans and is mentioned in a cookery book written in AD 230 by Apicius Caelius. Carrots were first brought to Britain during the reign of Elizabeth I, by Flemish refugees. In those days some of our now-familiar vegetables were luxuries but, following their successful cultivation in Kent, carrots quickly spread to other parts of the country. During the reign of James I, fashionable ladies wore the fernlike leaves in their hair as ornamentation.

Packeted seeds are available from plant nurseries and gardening centres. The vegetables are available throughout the year from greengrocers' and market stalls.

Carrots are a rich source of vitamin A — vital for healthy skin — which is why they should play a very prominent part in every woman's beauty programme. When taken frequently, carrot juice from freshly grown vegetables is known to cure and prevent spots and blemishes and is good not only for the complexion, but the eyes and hair as well. It is a proven ingredient in certain facial masks and skin milks. However, certain plant and vegetable juices, including carrot juice, can be harmful if taken or used to excess, so be careful.

Cornflower (Centaurea cyanus)

Cornflowers were a favourite garden plant in Tudor times, and artists, most of whom were poor, extracted and treated the blue juice from the flowers, using it as a dye in their watercolours. The flower is considered lucky for anyone who beholds it, and is believed to have been the favourite of the German composer Beethoven.

This hardy and upright plant with greyish-green foliage may reach a height of three feet (90cm), and from early Summer to early Autumn produces round and brilliant blue blooms.

Cornflowers and poppies were a familiar sight in most British fields until a few years ago, when the modern pesticides killed them off. They can sometimes be seen growing wild on waste ground, and are still a very popular garden plant. Both the seeds and the young plants are sold in most horticultural centres, but, when buying them, do emphasize that you want the original all-blue variety, and not one of the hybrid strains!

Because the cornflower has a somewhat limited function in the field of natural beauty, one is quite wrongly inclined to write it off as being of little consequence. Yet all plants have their individual worth, and should never be underestimated. An infusion of cornflowers soothes and refreshes the mouth and brings a sparkle to tired eyes, and may be included in bath vinegars and mixed facial steaming treatments.

Cucumber (Cucumis sativus)

This deliciously cooling vegetable was widely used by the Ancient Greeks and Romans. Cultivated throughout the East, it was considered a delicacy. The Bible states that the Israelites in the wilderness complained to Moses of how they yearned for the Egyptian luxuries of 'cucumbers and melons'.

Cucumbers are thought to have originated in southern Asia. They were frequently seen in Britain during the fourteenth century, but for some reason their popularity waned and they had almost disappeared by the time Henry VIII ascended the throne, when they experienced a revival. It was not until the middle of the sixteenth century that cucumbers were cultivated on a wide scale.

A trailing annual, the plant is grown only for its fruit. The seeds or young plants are available from plant nurseries and gardening centres and the edible fruits are usually on sale in greengrocers' and supermarkets throughout the year. In the past, the value of cucumber as a beauty aid has been vastly underestimated. The pulp can be made into diverse cosmetics and, being so gentle, may be used on many sensitive skins. As an astringent or cleansing milk, it is difficult to better. During the Summer months, cucumber is invaluable for soothing and healing painful sunburn. It may be incorporated in a lotion to clear blemishes or used as a facial mask for minimizing enlarged pores and oiliness. Many commercially manufactured facial moisturizing creams, hand lotions and toilet soaps now include extract of cucumber, but you can make all of these yourself to suit your own individual requirements.

Eucalyptus (*Eucalyptus globulus*)

The German botanist and explorer, Baron Ferdinand von Müller, who was Director of Melbourne Botanical Gardens from 1857 to 1873, was the first to discover the wonderful antiseptic properties of eucalyptus, otherwise known as 'fever tree'. He noticed that the perfume resembled that of cajaput oil, and suggested that eucalyptus trees might help to rid marshland areas of fever. So, in 1857, seeds were planted in Algiers, where they flourished. This led to vast swampy districts being planted out with fever trees, the roots of which also have a valuable drying action on the surrounding land. The oil extracted from the leaves was widely used in Britain and other European countries during the late nineteenth century as a strong antiseptic to help cure bronchitis, whooping cough, typhoid, scarlet and other fevers.

The tree is very attractive, with bluish-green, ovate leaves, which turn to mid-green as they age. The bark, which is gradually shed each year, is bluish-white when newly exposed. A native of Tasmania, *Eucalyptus globulus* is frequently used in bedding out in public parks and gardens. It is also grown extensively in California and is not uncommon in Europe, parts of Africa, Australia and South America. Seeds and young shrubs are obtainable from plant nurseries and gardening centres, whilst dried eucalyptus leaves can be found in many herb shops.

Because of their marvellous antiseptic qualities, eucalyptus leaves may be used in a variety of beauty recipes. They can be made into a good sunburn remedy, a refreshing mouthwash, and are an ingredient of many bath gels and oils.

Fennel, garden fennel (*Foeniculum vulgare*)

The Ancient Greeks and Romans ate the strongly flavoured fennel seeds to give them strength, and during the reign of Edward I of England quantities of these seeds were consumed by rich and poor alike.

This aromatic perennial, with bluish-green feather-like foliage, produces clusters of brilliant yellow blooms in mid-Summer. Growing to a height of approximately five feet (1.5 metres), it can be seen either cultivated or wild, particularly on waste ground near the sea. Dried fennel seeds may be purchased from most delicatessens and health food shops. The growing plants are often available in the larger nurseries and gardening centres.

Apart from its medicinal and culinary uses, the seeds when chewed are good for sweetening the breath. An infusion of the seeds in water will soothe inflamed and swollen eyelids. The leaves are invaluable for deep-cleansing the pores of the skin with a face pack or facial steam treatment. Finally, to give your hair a boost, the leaves may be infused to make a marvellous herbal hair rinse.

Horseradish (Cochlearia armoracia)

The horseradish was first used by the Ancient Greeks as a medicinal plant for the relief of gout, sciatica and dropsy. By the mid-thirteenth century the Germans were making it into a sauce, and eating it as a condiment for fish and meat dishes, but unfortunately it was not until the sixteenth century that it eventually found its way to Britain. This long-lasting perennial, with its characteristic large and wavy leaves may reach a height of around two feet (60cm). However, it is not cultivated for either the rough foliage, or the small white flowers which appear in early Summer, but for its much valued long tap-root which, if not cut regularly, can prove more than a little invasive.

Horseradish may be seen thriving naturally in fields and waste ground throughout Europe. The roots, known as 'thongs', are frequently on sale at those horticultural and greengrocery establishments which specialize in herbs and different forms of 'seasoning' plants, particularly during the latter part of the Winter.

Those of you who feel that freckles mar rather than enhance your appearance, might like to try the Horseradish recipe on page 97. Horseradish may be used when treating acne and problem complexions, and can quickly and simply be transformed into a lovely skin freshener and nail whitening lotion.

Houseleek (Sempervivum tectorum)

This attractive succulent was often mentioned in the writings of the Ancient Greeks and Romans, for it was generally believed to guard against the ill-effects of storms by acting as a conductor of electricity. It was consequently displayed in vases outside many Roman houses. The Emperor Charlemagne, too, proclaimed that the roof of every household should be planted with some houseleeks and in Wales, even now, some people still practise this superstitious custom.

Houseleek is a distinctive and hardy evergreen that carries a rosette of fleshy green leaves, often flecked with reddish-brown. The small, rose-coloured daisy-like flowers form on tall stems in summer. An extremely common garden plant, houseleeks are grown in Britain and many parts of Europe. They are propagated by detaching the offsets, which are produced each year, and both the seeds and potted speciments are often available from plant nurseries and gardening centres.

The houseleek has long been valued as a wonderfully beneficial skin herb. It may be included in skin creams, lotions and facial steam treatments.

Lavender, Old English lavender (Lavendula spica)

The word *Lavendula* originates from the Latin word *lavo*, meaning to wash — possibly because lavender was used in the making of soap and many other toiletries. Indigenous to both Britain and the Mediterranean countries, the silver-leaved lavender produces long, fragrant, spiky bluish flowers throughout the summer and early autumn. The extremely common shrub is easily obtainable from gardening suppliers.

Lavender is one of the most accommodating of all herbs, for apart from its many medicinal uses it can be easily used to make a number of cosmetic aids. It makes an effective mouthwash, eye lotion, and skin tonic, it is included in certain soaps, and is an essential ingredient in some creams, hair rinses and colognes. As a bath additive it reigns supreme and other lotions, oils, vinegars and milks containing it all act as fragrant and beautifying skin cleansers.

Lettuce (Lactuca sativa)

Lettuce was grown by the Ancient Romans and the Greeks. Although we don't know exactly where it originated, both Siberia and the Mediterranean regions have been suggested. The much crisper and taller-growing cos lettuce, which was brought from the Greek Archipelago, is believed to have come from the island of Cos. Lettuce has been grown in Britain certainly since 1562 and perhaps even before. The pre-packed seeds are available from any gardening nursery, large or small, and the leafy plants are sold in supermarkets and greengrocery shops during most of the year.

Lettuce is frequently included in skin preparations. It is invaluable in gently soothing and curing skin that has been overexposed to the sun, wind or water, and I regularly make up a lettuce lotion for a facial tonic. Because it is rich in vitamins and contains remarkable cleansing properties it is a valuable ingredient in toilet soaps and facial cleansers.

Marigold, pot marigold, garden marigold (Calendula officinalis)

For hundreds of years the marigold has been valued as a healing plant. During the seventeenth century the fresh heads were plucked and used as an antiseptic to cleanse and relieve wounds, whilst the leaves were bruised and applied to reduce fevers. Settlers who emigrated to America took marigold seeds with them, and thus marigolds were available to soothe the wounds of soldiers injured during the American Civil War.

A native of southern Europe, marigold is a hardy annual that may be seen growing wild on wasteland and in fields. It is more often cultivated in gardens and public parks, where it blooms and seeds freely. The familiar flattish, brilliant orange flowers appear in late spring, normally opening only in daylight hours. In Germany, when marigolds fail to open by the morning it is considered by many to be a sign of forthcoming rain. Packeted seeds and young plants are obtainable from most gardening stores.

When infused in water, marigold blooms make a tea that, when sipped, tones up a lazy circulation. It is also said to alleviate varicose veins. Since the blooms have healing properties, the cooled infusion is valuable as a skin tonic for oily, blemished complexions., It can also be used as a rich skin moisturizer, a hair shampoo, and a rinse, the latter being particularly useful in highlighting the pretty tints in brown and reddish hair.

Parsley (Carum petroselinum)

The Greeks believed that parsley germinated from the spilled blood of Archemorus, who was a great hero of the time. The champions of the Isthmian games were crowned with garlands of parsley. The herb is thought to have been brought to England by the Romans, but there is little evidence of it being grown here until 1548.

The strain of parsley most frequently encountered today is *C.p. crispum*, a descendant of the original variety. A hardy biennial which is cultivated as an annual, it has brilliant green and curled foliage, and is a rich source of vitamin C. Umbels of greenish-yellow flowers are borne on short stalks in Summer. Plant nurseries and gardening centres sell either the seeds or the young plants. The freshly plucked foliage is available most of the year from supermarkets and greengrocers' shops.

I think that parsley is one of the most undervalued of all the raw materials for herbal beauty preparations. It makes an excellent rinse for dark hair and proves a good antidote for dandruff. Those who have a very oily skin might like to try the special parsley and lavender anti-acne skin food and the mint and parsley milk. This, if employed in conjunction with a weekly face mask, can produce remarkably good results. Parsley also makes good anti-freckle and eye lotions and an excellent mouthwash.

Peppermint (Mentha × piperita)

Peppermint, perhaps the most fragrant and best-known of all the mints, is believed to have been cultivated by the Ancient Egyptians. The Ancient Greeks also used it, adding sprays to their bath water in much the same way as we use essences, salts, and oils today. The Romans first brought it to Britain, using it both to decorate their dining tables and flavour their sauces. During the latter part of the seventeenth century, peppermint was widely cultivated in the London area.

The peppermint has serrated and hairy leaves tinged with red, and produces spiky lilac-coloured blooms between the axils of the upper leaves. The purplish stems may reach a height of nearly three feet (90cm) and can sometimes be seen growing naturally alongside rivers, ponds, and streams. Most herb-growers and nurseries keep a steady supply.

The oil extracted from the leaves is used commercially in the manufacture of toiletries and perfumes. I use it in both a cooling cologne and a rather special night cream. The leaves may be infused to make a tea, which may be taken either as a mild sedative or as an after-dinner stomach-settler. Once cooled, the tea becomes cosmetically useful as a moisturizer, often helping to banish blemishes. It can also be blended to make a refreshing complexion milk, hair rinse, bath vinegar or mouthwash.

Potato (*Solanum tuberosum*)

Our own European potato originates from the tuberous plant that was discovered by the Spaniards in the Andes during the early sixteenth century, but the South American Indians have been cooking and eating potatoes for well over two thousand years.

At first prejudice existed against the plant, because other members of this family, such as Mandrake, were associated with witchcraft. By the early 1600s the Irish were cultivating the potato, and it became the staple food of the poor. By the 1760s, potatoes were cultivated in many parts of Scotland, but it was not until later in the eighteenth century that the potato became the principal source of food for the poorer people of England.

These tuberous fruits require no description, but it must be remembered that any green parts of the potato, like the foliage, are poisonous and should never be eaten.

Apart from its use in cooking, the potato is effective in a number of beauty preparations. It can be quickly transformed into a wonderful hand lotion and facial cleanser suitable for both dry and normal complexions. Being gentle, it may be applied to swollen eyelids and to sunburn. Indeed, as a beauty aid it is versatile and far more valuable than is generally supposed.

Rhubarb (*Rheum rhaponticum*)

Rhubarb was practically unknown in the West until the early 1700s, when the well-known Dutch physician, Boerhaave, obtained some seeds from a Tartanian merchant. Once sown, they produced two very distinct species, the 'Garden Rhubarb' (*Rheum rhaponticum*) and the 'Turkey Rhubarb' (*R. palmatum*). Then, in 1777, an English apothecary from Oxfordshire decided to cultivate some seeds which he had received from Russia some fifteen years previously, and the resulting plants produced what was believed to be an effective drug of good quality. The rhubarb plantations in Banbury are still in existence today, and there his descendants continue in the family tradition of growing varying strains of rhubarb, including the *R. officinale*, which first made its appearance in Britain in 1873.

A hardy perennial, it is grown solely for its thick red edible stems, which appear almost continuously from late Winter to mid-Summer. However, the huge leaves which top the stalks like giant Indian honorific parasols, are extremely poisonous, and should never be taken internally under any circumstances.

The edible stems are available from greengrocers for approximately six months of the year. Young plants are usually purchased from plant nurseries and garden supply centres. Although seeds may also be purchased, this form of propagation often results in only weak and inferior stock, which will take several years before it is ready to crop.

There are many vegetable colourings which are used to gently and effectively dye the hair, and rhubarb is just one of them. Whether you have fair, light or dark brown hair, the root or sticks may be used to enliven it with a rich and natural golden look!

Rose (Rosa)

The rose is a symbol of love and purity, and the leaves were once scattered at weddings just as we throw confetti today for good luck.

The first cultivated roses were red and probably originated in northern Persia. They spread to Greece, and in some Greek towns today visitors are still offered rose jam when taking refreshments. The Romans used roses extensively, and a rose suspended above the table signified that all confidences were to remain secrets afterwards. Hence the often ornate ceiling decorations in more modern rooms are known as roses.

The discovery of otto or oil of roses in the late sixteenth or early seventeenth century was made during the wedding feast of the Princess Nair-Djihan and the Emperor Djihanguyr. As part of the celebrations, a deep trench had been dug around the garden and filled with rosewater. When the young couple came to row on its scented surface, they noticed that the sun had caused the essential oil to separate from the water. When a film of this oil was removed, it was found to have a highly concentrated perfume. By 1612, otto of roses was being manufactured in large quantities at Shiraz in Persia.

No general description could possibly cover the hundreds of different roses but the often brilliantly coloureds heads are familiar to all. The shrubs are easily purchased from plant nurseries and gardening centres.

The perfume from rose petals is extracted to make either rosewater or otto of roses, and, cosmetically, either makes a highly perfumed skin softener. Both are included in various colognes and toilet waters, face creams, hand lotions and shampoos. Rosewater is both an excellent mouthwash and a soothing and gentle remedy for chapped, cracked and rough skin, whilst the oil makes a rich and luxuriously perfumed bath essence.

Rosemary, compass weed, polar plant (Rosmarinus officinalis)

In ancient Greece, students wore sprays of rosemary in their hair because it was believed that it improved the memory! The first known rosemary plants arrived in Britain in the 1300s, sent by the Countess of Hainault to her daughter who was Queen to Edward III.

By the fifteenth century, the herb was widely cultivated and was used as a cheaper substitute for incense. It was also included in a number of everyday tonics and remedies.

A native of Asia Minor and southern Europe, this erect shrub has mid-green leathery leaves, whose undersides are covered with fine, white hairs. The lilac-coloured flowers open in early spring and continue blooming intermittently until early autumn. When left to grow in the wild, the shrubs often prefer coastal districts — not surprisingly perhaps, since its generic name *Rosmarinus* is derived from the Latin words *ros* (dew) and *marinus* (maritime). Dried rosemary is a common culinary herb, which may be purchased easily. Growing plants are sold in many of the larger nurseries and garden centres.

Rosemary has long been an ingredient of eau de cologne and many hair preparations. It can be made into an effective remedy for dandruff, which, as a marvellous hair rinse and tonic, leaves the hair shining with health and can be made at home. Rosemary also makes a good facial steam treatment, bath additive and foot bath.

Sage, red sage, garden sage (*Salvia officinalis*)

The leaves of garden sage have been employed in many ways for thousands of years, and both Theophrastus and Pliny detailed and praised their virtues. The Romans called sage *herb sacra*, believing that it was to be revered, and used it to encourage conception, as a general tonic and as a remedy for a number of ills. It was also a firm favourite with the Chinese.

First known as 'sawge' in this country, sage was considered an essential garden plant by the seventeenth century. Our ancestors brewed the leaves and consumed the herbal tea as an everyday drink long before the Indian beverage had been heard of in Britain. The leaves were also used to whiten the teeth and strengthen the gums, a practice which continues today.

Salvia officinalis is a perennial with oval and greyish-green, wrinkled foliage. The bluish-violet blooms appear at any time from early to mid-Summer. The seeds and growing plants are on sale at the usual sources during most of the year and the dried herbs may be found in most food shops.

Sage, with its vibrant flavour, is a constituent of gargles. The oil extracted from the plant is used in the manufacture of soaps and perfumes. At home this herb may be used to make a variety of bath mixes, colognes, mouthwashes, toothpastes and lip creams. Used in shampoos, it stimulates the scalp. It also offers a subtle means of darkening greying hair.

Southernwood (*Artemisia abrotanum*)

The Southernwood has been cultivated as a medicinal plant throughout the Mediterranean countries since Roman times, but it did not reach Britain until 1548.

People scattered it in bedrooms because it was thought to be an aphrodisiac. When women walked to church, they often carried large posies of southernwood to prevent them from falling asleep during the seemingly interminable sermons. When prisoners appeared in court, sprays of the plant were placed in the dock next to them to protect others from the fevers that afflicted many of these unfortunates.

A semi-evergreen shrub, southernwood has small, greyish-green, divided foliage. During the summer it has clusters of tiny yellow blooms. As a garden plant it grows throughout Southern Europe. Potted specimens are obtainable from many plant nurseries and gardening centres and the dried leaves are sold in many herb shops.

Southernwood makes a toning bath additive but is more often used as a hair rinse or tonic.

Strawberry (Fragaria × ananassa)

Strawberries were mentioned in some early English manuscripts of the tenth century, and yet it took another seven hundred years before Europe sampled the first cultivated fruits. These were known as 'Little Scarlet', or 'Scarlet Woodland' strawberry (*F. virginiana*), and they arrived from Virginia in 1629. Later another strain, the 'West Coast Pine' strawberry (*F. chiloensis*), was also imported. In Europe, cross-breeding quickly resulted in the improved hybrid varieties of the nineteenth century.

Today's strawberries thrive from early Summer to Autumn but exactly when they fruit depends on the individual strain. Adult plants perpetuate the species by producing characteristic runners, which if left untended quickly put down roots and grow independently. Seeds and young plants are available from plant nurseries and gardening centres. The fruit can be seen in greengrocery shops and fruit stalls throughout the summer.

A badly sunburned face or back is extremely painful and many people cannot bear the application of any cream, however soothing it may prove to be. Yet a little strawberry sunburn splash immediately provides relief. Strawberries also make a marvellously effective, as well as mouth-watering, teeth whitener. Try them also in a face mask, a fruity astringent water and strawberry complexion milk.

Thyme, garden thyme (Thymus vulgaris)

Few kitchens are without this particular herb, but it has long been appreciated too for its antiseptic qualities. In both the Crimean and First World Wars, it was used to soothe and disinfect the wounds of injured soldiers. The Ancient Romans put it in their baths. It was they who first introduced it to Britain, where it has been widely cultivated since the 1400s. Thyme is a dwarf evergreen shrub, with characteristic deep green, aromatic leaves, and it bears clusters of mauve flowers from the leaf axils in early summer. These flowers eventually produce a multitude of small seeds. Thyme can be very easily purchased either in seed form or as young plants. The dried and crushed leaves are usually found in health shops and food stores.

Thyme is still used in manufactured soaps and antiseptics, and it can play a vital role in many home-made toiletries. It makes a cooling facial tonic and astringent, a relaxing footbath and ordinary bath additive, and a wonderful herbal shampoo.

Tomato (*Lycopersicon esculentum*)

The tomato was originally known as the 'Peruvian golden' or 'love apple'. It arrived in Italy during the sixteenth century. These tender and half-hardy annuals can be cultivated under glass and out of doors, and they are grown entirely for the familiar crop of fruits. These are sold by greengrocers all the year round, while potted seedlings are plentiful in plant nurseries and garden centres.

Tomatoes can be very messy and sticky when used in making toiletries. However, the tomato recipes in this book are designed to be as pure and pleasing as possible.

People with unsightly, enlarged pores should regularly treat themselves to a tomato face mask. Indeed, anyone with either an extremely oily or a very dry skin will certainly benefit from this treatment. Once delighted with the results, you will want to try the tomato skin tonic and hand lotion as well.

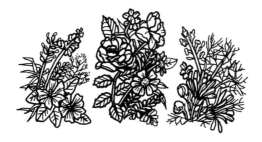

5

In the Wild

Birch (Betula alba/pendula)

The silver birch is still considered a protection against evil spirits by some people in northern Europe. The small and ovate mid-green leaves are borne on trailing branches. In summer the larger male catkins appear from the tips of the newly sprouted shoots, whilst the smaller, green female ones are set much further back. This lovely tree is always recognizable by its extremely beautiful silvery-white bark. Birch trees are so ornamental and freely germinating that they can be found growing in private gardens, public parks, woodlands and waste ground. There should be no difficulty in obtaining a supply of fresh leaves when they are in season. Dried leaves can also be purchased from herbal shops.

I am always experimenting with new herbal hair recipes, and I have used birch leaves in a selection of shampoos, conditioning lotions and rinses. They also help to produce a delightful and effective skin lotion.

Camomile, Chamomile (Chamaemelum nobile)

The name 'camomile' or 'chamomile' is derived from the Greek word *chamaimelon — chamai*, meaning 'on the ground', and *melon* meaning 'apple'. This latter word refers, of course, to *camomile's* apple-like fragrance.

The plant was used widely by the Ancient Egyptians for its healing qualities. It is believed to have been used in England as early as 1265. During the late nineteenth century, this herb was grown in large quantities at Mitcham in Surrey purely for its medicinal properties. Although it is still cultivated in several European countries, it is now produced almost solely for its oil, which is extracted and used in modern hair shampoos.

44

A low-growing perennial, camomile looks somewhat like moss. The yellow and white daisy-like flowers, which are borne on leafless stems, appear from early to late Summer. A native of Britain and Europe, it may be seen growing wild on heath and wasteland and should not be difficult to obtain.

Camomile is extremely versatile as a beauty aid. As well as improving and highlighting fair hair, it is effective in helping acne and soothing tired eyes and chapped hands. It makes a good skin cleanser and astringent and can be made into a number of bath soaks, soaps and all-over body splashes.

Clover (*Trifolium pratense — red; Trifolium repens — white*)

To the Anglo-Saxons, red clover, which they referred to as 'Claefra', was essentially a medicinal herb, and later on our ancestors included it in potions to cure bronchitis and chest colds. For hundreds of years it was considered a safeguard against witchcraft and evil spirits.

The white clover is a native of central and northern Asia and Europe, including Britain, and it grows abundantly throughout the U.S.A. Originally, it was called 'Clafre', which became changed down the ages to 'claver' and ultimately 'clover'. The clovers, with their familiar three-leaved foliage, and red or white pom-pom like blooms, reproduce by means of creeping runners, and are so well known that they need no further description.

The red variety can often be found growing in meadows, where it is considered a valuable cattle fodder. However, it is rarely seen in gardens, because of its natural aversion to chemically fertilized soils. The white strain has no such aversion and, apart from being a familiar wasteland flower, it is sometimes cultivated as a lawn.

The dried heads of the red clover are sold at most good herbal shops. They make a lovely soothing lip-salve, whilst the white blossoms are effective in safely bleaching unsightly freckles. Both varieties can be used either separately or together, to produce a 'heady' hair rinse.

Comfrey (*Symphytum officinale*)

Since the Middle Ages, comfrey has been considered primarily as a healing plant, and for very good reason too, as we shall see. The name itself derived from the word 'con-firma', and refers to the use made of comfrey in the aiding and mending of broken bones. (Other names for comfrey include Knit Bone, Boneset and Knitback.) The treatment, which has been practised for many hundreds of years, at first counted the majority of the medical fraternity among its detractors. That was still the situation until fairly recently. Greater acceptance came when comfrey was found to contain exceptionally high proportions of silica and alantoin, both of which are necessary to the successful healing of such injuries.

The perennial comfrey with long, wavy-edged, and hairy leaves, may reach a height of three feet (90cm). The small bell-like flowers which range in colour from cream to pink, blue or lilac, bloom throughout the Summer.

The Borage family embraces this plant, which may be found occasionally in nurseries which specialize in a wide range of all-purpose herbs. However, a native of Europe and some parts of Asia, it is more likely to be found growing wild alongside rivers, pools and streams.

Those of you who eat and drink only those things which are considered utterly pure will be pleased to learn that the ground roots of comfrey, combined with those of dandelion and chicory, make a good vegetable substitute for the ordinary and more harmful types of conventional coffee. Once extracted, the comfrey oil may be blended in a wonderfully healing and beautifying bath mixture. Alternatively, the plant itself may be used as a more simple bathing additive. Toilet soaps, hair rinses, and hand creams are also enhanced by the inclusion of comfrey, the latter being marvellous for those who, until now, have suffered from sore and chapped hands.

Cowslip (*Primula veris*)

The word 'cowslip' comes from the Anglo-Saxon 'cuslippe', yet in some country districts it is still occasionally referred to as 'paigles' which means 'St Peter', because it was supposed to represent the Keys of Heaven which St Peter holds. Many of the famous herbalists of different periods, such as Pliny, Gerard and Culpeper, used the flowers, leaves and roots to treat nervous disorders, skin complaints, cramp, vertigo and convulsions.

The cowslip bears clusters of downy wrinkled foliage and during the early Spring grows a single stem which produces umbels of sweetly perfumed, creamy yellow flowers. This fairly common plant grows wild on mainly chalky soil throughout Europe, North America, China and Japan.

As a facial herb, cowslip flowers are marvellous when added to skin creams and sunburn lotions. They have a slightly bleaching effect and the skin lotion also has a really deep cleansing action. Cowslip blooms also make a wonderfully luxurious and relaxing bath ingredient, but it is best to treat yourself to a slow and pampering soak if you are to derive full benefit.

Dandelion (*Taraxacum officinale*)

As early as the tenth century, Arabian physicians and herbalists were writing about the diuretic effects of the dandelion, which was referred to as a wild endive. Three hundred years later many Welsh medicines contained it. In England during the reign of Queen Victoria, it was grown in most gardens as a salad vegetable. Sometimes called 'Lion's Tooth' (*dent de lion*) because of its serrated and molar like leaves, it is today cultivated in India and the U.S.A. as a cure for liver complaints. Throughout Europe it is a widely accepted ingredient of many tonics and patent medicines.

This stemless plant is composed of a tapering tap-root and green serrated leaves, both of which exude a milky juice when cut. From early Spring until Autumn, the dandelion bears brilliant yellow, flat-topped flowers. The dandelion can be found growing wild almost everywhere, so most people should find it very easy to obtain a regular supply of leaves and roots. If you live in a city, both leaves and roots are obtainable from better herb shops.

Dandelion leaves make a good cleansing and moisturizing milk and face mask, both of which are particularly suited to those who have sallow complexions. When used with other ingredients in bath water, they can sometimes help those who are trying to lose weight.

Elder (Sambucus nigra)

Legend has it that Judas Iscariot was hung from gallows made of elder and that the cross on which Christ died was of the same wood. So it is understandable that this shrub became a symbol of death and was never used in the construction of such things as baby cradles. The Romans employed various parts of the elder bush in the making of medicines. The berries were used as a black hair dye and this has continued through to modern times.

The shrub may reach a height of around thirty-two feet (10 metres), although specimens of half that size are more usual. It has dark green pinnate leaves and greyish-green bark, but it is the flowers that are distinctive. These creamy white, flattened blooms appear in mid-Summer and are followed in early Autumn by clusters of small, black berries. One doesn't have to travel far to find elder growing in gardens, woods and wasteland where the blossoms and berries may be gathered quite freely. Packeted dried flowers are available throughout the year from herb shops.

Elderflower water has been a popular and important beauty aid for centuries and is often included in hand lotions and nourishing and cleansing creams or milks. It also makes a gentle and soothing eyebath for strained and tired eyes. As a lotion it improves enlarged pores and spotty complexions. Used regularly, it helps to bleach freckles.

Golden Seal (Hydrastis canadensis)

The American Indians used this herb both as a medicine and as a yellow dye, and apparently extolled its virtues to the early American settlers. As a result this common wild plant became so much sought after that it is now extinct in many American states. A member of the buttercup family, it was first introduced to Britain in 1760 and was later grown in the botanical gardens at Kew, Dublin and Edinburgh. Eventually it was accepted as a genuine pharmaceutical herb.

Golden seal is a perennial with dark-green and prominently veined hairy leaves, and a brilliant yellow, horizontal-growing root-stock. In early Spring it produces small greenish-white flowers, and these are followed in the Summer by red, raspberry-like fruits.

As well as being cultivated in certain states the plant grows wild in parts of North America;

the root is dried and exported to many countries including Britain, where it is sold in health shops.

Golden Seal is a mild and gentle cleansing herb, used in eye lotions, tooth powders, and mouthwashes. All of these can be produced at home.

Groundsel *(Senecio vulgaris)*

Pliny prescribed grounsel for toothache; later the Anglo-Saxons used it as a multi-purpose healing herb. By the fifteenth century groundsel was grown extensively with other medicinal plants in many monastery gardens. The women of the Scottish Highlands used to wear pieces of the root around their necks as a guard against the ague and all forms of evil witchcraft. When covered with boiling water, groundsel acts as a water softener and it is included in some patented eye lotions.

This ragged-looking annual (and biennial) has feathery lobed, dark-green leaves. Throughout most of the Spring and Summer it bears small yellow flowers. A common plant, groundsel can be found growing freely in untended gardens, fields and wasteland areas throughout Europe and parts of Asia.

Groundsel is gentle and healing. Those with chapped hands should try coating them in my special groundsel lotion. Indeed, groundsel is so safe that it can even be recommended for treating swollen eyes. When you want to look your best, but don't because your eyes are tired, give yourself a groundsel eye pack.

Horsetail *(Equisetum arvense)*

In Ancient Rome, horsetail leaves were crushed and applied to wounds to ease and stop bleeding. In the seventeenth century, horsetail was used both as a medicinal herb and as a practical means of polishing pewter — hence its popular name, 'scouring rush'. In China and some other countries it is still harvested and sold for a variety of medicinal purposes.

This invasive and completely flowerless plant looks spiky — somewhat like a tiny skeleton pine tree from which all the needles have fallen. Indigenous to many European countries including Britain, it flourishes in those gardens, fields and wastelands where the soil is not chalky. The herb is commercially harvested, dried and sold in good health and herbal shops.

Horsetail is an essential ingredient in certain herbal splashes and hair rinses. An astringent skin lotion made from horsetail may prove helpful to those with enlarged pores, while an infusion of horsetail helps to strengthen flaking and brittle nails.

Lady's Bedstraw *(Galium verum)*

The name of this plant could well allude to the Virgin Mary as the plant is believed to be one of those which were used to line the cradle of the newly-born Christ.

The herb has been used for centuries to curdle milk and to impart a good colour to the resulting cheeses; in Gloucester, both lady's bedstraw and nettle are used. The plant's generic name, *Galium*, comes from the Greek word *gala*, meaning 'milk', In sixteenth-century England, it was referred to as 'cheese rennet'. During the reign of Henry VIII, women coloured their hair with it. The yellow dye extracted from the stems and leaves and the red obtained from the roots are widely used in parts of Ireland today.

Lady's bedstraw is a perennial with whorls of narrow leaves, the stems of which may reach two feet (60cm) in height. Throughout the Summer it produces clusters of brilliant yellow flowers. It grows profusely in fields, on banks and in meadows.

Tired ankles and feet respond quickly to a soaking in an infusion of lady's bedstraw.

Lime (Tilia × europaea)

Also known as the linden, common lime or linn tree, the flowers from this handsome tree were scattered by the Vikings in the bridal chambers of newly married couples to ensure that they would produce children similarly tall and handsome.

The sweet-perfumed, smooth-barked lime tree grows to a height of around thirty feet (9 metres). In Summer, from beneath its mid-green, heart-shaped leaves hang clusters of yellowish-white flowers. The blooms contain an abundance of sweet nectar, from which bees produce the finest of all honey. Lindens grow naturally in most parts of Europe and Great Britain. They are also cultivated, especially in parks and public gardens.

An infusion of the dried flowers is taken in some parts of Europe as a cure for indigestion and headaches. It is better known, however, for its calming effects — a bath in which lime flowers have been steeped encourages restful sleep. As a beautifier, the fresh flowers make a wonderful hair tonic, hair rinse and facial steam treatment. Women who wish safely to lighten their complexions, bleach freckles or minimize wrinkles may be helped by the natural properties of lime flowers.

Marshmallow (Althaea officinalis)

In 287 BC Theophrastus compiled a list of several hundred plants and their therapeutic uses. Of all these, one of the most important was the marshmallow. It is believed to have been introduced into England by the Romans, who ate it as a vegetable and thought it a great delicacy.

The Greeks prepared the seeds in oil and served them as a general tonic and health-giving food. The generic name, *Althaea,* is derived from the Greek word *altho*, meaning 'to cure'.

Marshmallow has greyish-green serrated foliage and may reach a height of approximately six feet (1.8 metres). From early summer to early autumn this perennial produces light pink, five-petalled blooms. *Althaea officinalis* grows by ponds, rivers and streams. It is found throughout Europe including Britain, and in many parts of the U.S.A. Both the dried roots and leaves may be purchased from health shops.

Because of its well-known skin-softening qualities, the dried root is made into a number of skin lotions and creams, all of which are superb for extra-sensitive skins. The leaves, when steeped in water, produce a liquid that serves as a soothing lotion for strained and inflamed eyes.

Mullein (Verbascum thapsus)

The Ancient Romans dipped the downy mullein leaves and stems into tallow and used them as tapers. The women soon discovered that an effective hair dye could be obtained by first infusing the yellow flowers and then using the strained liquid as a golden hair rinse. Poor people stuffed the crushed leaves into their stockings to help keep their feet and legs warm. Long before the introduction of cotton into Britain, mullein plants were dried for use as lamp wicks, and this is why the plant is sometimes still referred to as 'candlewick plant'.

Mullein is a biennial with large greyish-green foliage and many grow six feet (1.8 metres) tall. The yellow flowers form in closely grouped, club-shaped clusters and appear throughout the Summer. Mullein is a fairly common plant, to be found growing naturally on waste ground and alongside road verges in Asia, Europe and North America. It is also harvested commercially, dried and then sold in good herb shops.

Like Roman women of long ago, you might like to experiment with this safe and completely natural golden hair colourant.

Nettle (Urtica dioica)

The word nettle comes from the Anglo-Saxon word 'noedl', meaning 'needle' — referring to the plant's defensive and often painful sting. Nettle has an extremely high vitamin C content, and has long been used in tonics and medicines and eaten as a cooked green vegetable.

A perennial with a creeping rootstock and erect stems, it grows to a height of five feet (1.5 metres) when provided with good growing conditions. On the stem it has pairs of hairy, toothed and dark-green leaves. Nettle grows plentifully on any rich waste ground. The dried leaves are always available in health shops.

As yet, few people realize the immense worth of this so-called weed, despite it being an important part of many natural beauty preparations. As a general hair rinse, tonic and conditioner it cannot be bettered, and it can be used daily to keep the hair strong, healthy and free from dandruff. I also add a nettle infusion to many of my own hair shampoos. Furthermore it makes a fine skin tonic and bath soak. Finally at the end of a particularly exhausting day, when your feet are really tired soak them in a foot-bath of warm, nettle-steeped water.

Pine (*Pinus*)

The name Virgil used for this tree is *pinus*, which might well have been derived from the word *picis* or *pix*, referring to the resin exuded from these particular trees.

Any of the many pines may be used cosmetically, for they all possess the same woodland fragrance. They can be found growing together or singly in vast forests throughout the northern hemisphere.

The pine needles are the raw material for a number of hair lotions and bath ingredients, including, of course, the rich and highly recommended pine gel and bath soak.

Soapwort (*Saponaria officinalis*)

The family name *Saponaria* comes from the Latin word *sapo*, meaning 'soap', and this plant was the original soap. People washed both themselves and their clothes by crushing and boiling the leaves, which lathered and removed dirt and grease relatively easily.

Also referred to as 'latherwort', 'crow-soap', 'bruisewort' and 'soaproot', this hardy annual can reach a height of four feet (1.2 metres). The broad, elliptical leaves form opposite each other, and from early Summer to Autumn, the plant bears clusters of large pink flower heads. Soapwort may be found growing in hedgerows and wasteland. The dried herbs are obtainable from health shops.

As a cosmetic herb, soapwort is popular in bath gels and shampoos, as it affords a pure, natural and invigorating way of washing your body and hair. In the chapter on Hair, I include my own favourite high-protein shampoo (see page 125).

Valerian (*Valeriana officinalis*)

In medieval times Valerian was believed to cure most of the common maladies. The Anglo-Saxons ate it as a salad vegetable, and it is first mentioned in medical writings of the ninth and tenth centuries. At this period it was used to treat insomnia and other nervous disorders. By 1568 it was used in many medicines and perfumes; it had become an everyday custom to place the sweet-smelling roots amongst clothes so that they would absorb the perfume as our parents' linen absorbed lavender.

Just twenty-four years later, the intelligent and progressive Fabius Calumna treated himself with valerian and thus cured himself of epilepsy. He made his detailed findings famous, which is why valerian is still used today.

Bright green leaves form in pairs up the medium tall stems, which can reach a height of four feet (1.2 metres). Clusters of fluffy, pale-pink flowers appear in late Spring and early Summer. Valerian is frequently to be found growing wild in damp roadside ditches, marsh and wasteland in Britain. The root, which is the only part used, is grown commercially on a large scale and sold in many health shops.

Those who are highly strung, or sleep badly, should try soaking in my soothing bath mixture just before going to bed. This is a safer and far more pleasant way of ensuring a sound night's sleep than taking sleeping pills. And a good night's sleep is a beautifier in itself! A skin lotion distilled from the root is a marvellous cure for sore rashes and spots.

Common or White Willow *(Salix alba)*

It was under the willow trees of Babylon that the captured children of Israel wept for their homeland, and because of this sad story these trees have sometimes been considered a symbol of grief. Yet in China the willow is indicative of eternal life. There, coffins are covered with sprays of willow and, after burial, young willow saplings are planted alongside the graves, to ensure that the souls of the newly departed remain immortal.

Until the early part of the twentieth century, the only source of the medicinal salicylic acid, and its derivative, aspirin, was the bark of the willow. This was also used in the treatment of rheumatism.

An elegant tree which may reach a height of forty feet (12 metres), the willow has tapering greyish-green foliage which appears with the catkins around late Spring. The willow is quite common in many parts of Britain. The bark can be bought from herb and health shops. Willow leaves make an excellent shampoo and a conditioning tonic. The bark is particularly effective in eliminating dandruff and is also a safe means of darkening grey hair.

Yarrow *(Achillea millefolium)*

This plant was supposed to have sprung from the whittlings of Achilles' spear whilst, somewhat less fancifully, another legend tells of Achilles using the herb to staunch the bleeding of his wounded soldiers. From these connections with the famous Greek hero is derived the yarrow's generic name, *Achillea*.

Down the ages, the yarrow has been highly regarded for its healing properties. By the mid-fifteenth century, it was extensively grown in most English gardens as a cure for fevers, colds, ulcers, sores and all sorts of inflammations — including toothache. It was also used on the skin and as a hair wash to allay baldness. By the seventeenth century it was consumed both raw and as a cooked vegetable.

This erect perennial has deeply cut, feathery foliage. Its rough-textured stalks may reach a height of twenty inches (50cm) and support clusters of flat-topped white or pink daisy-like flowers throughout the Summer. Yarrow can be found growing wild in fields, hedgerows and on waste ground. The dried herb is obtainable from herbalists and health shops.

Yarrow is effective in a range of cosmetics. It makes a superb cleansing lotion for greasy complexions, and those who suffer from oily hair will greatly appreciate the yarrow hair rinse. It makes excellent hair tonics and anti-dandruff and herbal shampoos, and is particularly beneficial when incorporated in face masks. It will soothe and soften chapped hands.

6

In the Kitchen Cupboard

Almond *(Prunus dulcis)*

Almonds were not cultivated in Britain until the sixteenth century — and even then it was purely for their glorious blossom. In Europe during the Middle Ages, the nuts were widely eaten — as can be seen from the household accounts of the Queen of France, Jeanne d'Evreux, which show that her establishment used 500 pounds (227 kilos) in 1372! Salted almonds became popular, possibly because of the belief that they prevented one from becoming drunk.

A romantic but tragic legend built up around the origin of the tree, concerning a young and lovely Thracian queen, Phyllis, and a noble called Demophoon, who fell in love and married. Soon after the ceremony the young man was summoned to Athens by the death of his father, but he promised to return within a month. When he failed to do so, the heartbroken bride died of grief and was transformed into an almond tree. When the wandering husband at last returned and discovered the terrible truth, he ran to embrace the leafless tree, which expressed his dead wife's undying love by immediately bursting into bloom!

The almond is widely cultivated throughout the Mediterranean, reaching a height of twenty-five feet (7.6 metres). The lovely and very characteristic pink flowers always appear before the leaves, and are later followed by the soft-coated fruits.

Almond oil is one of the oldest of all cosmetics and has been used by many famous beauties. It has proved so valuable that it is still one of the leading ingredients in a varied range of commercial preparations. There are home-made cosmetics for every skin need. You can eliminate blemishes, blackheads and enlarged pores from a neglected complexion by using almond face scrubs and masks. If your skin is sun-parched and flaky, refine and moisturize it with enriching almond balms and creams. Only very few women have completely flawless complexions, and even these must be cleansed daily and cared for.

Alum

Alum, known as either 'dried alum' or 'burned alum', is a crystalline solution of aluminium and potassium salts. When heated, the water evaporates leaving odourless white or yellowish granules. They are soluble in both hot and cold water. Alum is on sale in chemists' shops.

The solution may be used in a variety of astringents and skin tonics. It can be included in face creams and bath mixtures.

Apple (Malus)

Apples were cultivated in large quantities well before the Normal Conquest. Glastonbury was generally referred to as the 'apple orchard' and in many towns the early Saxons established completely separate markets in which to buy and sell apples. The Druids had a great respect for the fruit and cut their divining rods from the boughs of apple trees. Throughout the counties of England, there are many festivals on Christmas Eve called 'wassailing' which honour the apple.

The hardy, deciduous apple tree produces pinkish-white blossoms during the Spring, followed in the Summer and Autumn by the fruits. There are many species in Britain alone.

Apples are one of the oldest of all beauty aids — as many germs cannot survive in the presence of apple juice. This makes apples an obvious ingredient in hair rinses, skin tonics, masks and facials. They make a lovely contribution to handcreams.

Apricot (Prunus armeniaca)

Confucius wrote in the peaceful surroundings of a Chinese apricot grove, and when his work was completed he gave thanks by erecting an altar. The apricot originated in northern China and central Asia. It first appeared in Britain during the reign of Henry VIII. The tree has gnarled red branches and deep green leaves. It reaches a height of thirty feet (9 metres) when left to grow in the wild. In the Spring it bears pinkish-white blossom. Fresh apricots are only available from fruiterers when in season, although the dried and tinned fruit can always be found in supermarkets and health shops. The extracted oil is sold in chemists', herb and health shops.

Both fresh and dried apricots contain large amounts of vitamin A, which enriches, heals and revitalizes the skin. Being rich in polyunsaturated oils, the fruit makes first-class facial masks and body oils. The oil is particularly valuable, helping to erase stretch marks and wrinkles. I have included an all-purpose body oil, a face anti-wrinkle food and a neck cream in the recipe section of this book.

Avocado (Persea americana and Persea gratissima)

The avocado has been known for at least four hundred years. South American and Mexican women use it as a moisturizer to protect their skins from the hot and drying climate. It contains more protein than almost any other fruit. The oil content of the cultivated varieties can be as high as twenty-five per cent. It is extracted by peeling and de-seeding the fruit, cutting them into small sections and squeezing out the juice mechanically into enormous tanks. The oil is then refined.

The tree is a native of tropical and central America and of California and Florida, and may reach a height of thirty feet (9 metres). It has large, oval, deep-green leaves, and, although it flowers during its sixth year, it often proves fruitless until the seventh, when it starts to produce the thick-skinned, pear-shaped green fruits. The fresh fruits are on sale for most of the year from greengrocers and delicatessens. The oil, though not quite so readily available, may be found in herb and health shops, and may be ordered either from your chemist or from an aromatic oil company.

Avocados are rich in natural oil, protein, and vitamins A and B, and possess both 'penetrating' and 'keeping' qualities. They are thus particularly effective in nourishing creams. They have healing properties too, and contain lecithin, a protein which is excellent for conditioning dry and damaged hair, and for use in cleansing creams and masks.

Banana (*Musa sapientum*)

The banana is not really a tree, as is generally presumed, but an enormous plant. Ancient legend has it that when Eve successfully tempted Adam to take of the fruit in the Garden of Eden, it was the banana and not the apple that he ate.

The banana plant is a periennial which is nearly as broad as it is tall; in the warm climates of the Canary Islands, the Caribbean and south-east Asia it reaches heights of around seven feet (2 metres). The thick, brilliant green foliage can be over three feet (90cm) in length. The leaves form a canopy over the purplish, leathery bracts which encase the white blooms in mid-Summer. These are later followed by the long and seedless, green and yellow fruits.

Bananas are rich in vitamin A and potassium, and contain no substances to aggravate even the most sensitive skin. The fruit makes extremely good refining and cleansing masks.

Beer

Ancient clay tablets which have been discovered dating back to 6000 BC, describe the making of ale, that is beer made without hops. Hops have grown wild in England for centuries, but it was only during the Hundred Years War, 1337–1453, that the English soldiers first sampled and preferred the tasty Flanders beer made from hops — which is no doubt why hops were being cultivated in this country in 1523.

A beer hair shampoo I make myself is better than the manufactured brands — and much cheaper. It leaves hair looking clean and lustrous, without making it 'fly-away'. The 'body' that beer provides makes it valuable as a hair rinse and setting lotion.

Beeswax

Beeswax is a yellow wax, secreted by glands in the underside of bees, which the insects use to make the celled walls of the honeycomb. It takes an incredible eight pounds of honey to extract a single pound of beeswax! The wax is obtained by submerging the honeycomb in hot water and then straining off the slowly forming waxy liquid. White beeswax is prepared by bleaching the raw yellowish wax for extended periods in the sun and then treating it with acids. Tubs or jars of these two waxes are obtainable from chemists' and health shops.

Beeswax acts as an emulsifying agent and is an ingredient of many cleansing and all-purpose moisturizing creams. I have used it in several creams which both feed and perfume the skin.

Benzoin (Styrax benzoin)

The styrax tree was highly regarded by Pliny, and in the ancient past the gum from the tree was used to perfume scents, colognes, pomanders, washing balls and bracelets. Now it is more frequently to be found in Eastern mosques, where it is burned as a fragrant incense.

The styrax tree is deciduous, has pale green foliage, and may reach a height of around twenty feet (6 metres). Small white flowers appear during the middle and late Spring, followed by tiny green fruits, the seeds of which are often made into rosary beads. The tincture is obtainable from chemists but the gum is more likely to be found in the larger herb shops.

Both tincture and gum possess valuable antiseptic and preserving qualities, the gum sometimes being used in preference to the tincture because of its perfume and ability to bind ingredients together. Both are incorporated in many facial washes, masks, astringents, tonics, moisturizing and cleansing creams.

Borax (Sodium tetraborate)

Sodium tetraborate, or borax, is not a man-made chemical substance as one might suppose, but a natural product found on alkaline lake shores. Gently cleansing and slightly astringent, it is available in colourless powder, granule or crystal forms. Borax may be purchased from chemists, supermarkets and health shops.

Being only mildly alkaline, borax doesn't dry the skin and so may be used in a wide range of exciting and useful toiletries. There are soap substitutes and cleansing washes for all those who dislike using hard soap, plus bath mixtures, hair shampoos and lotions, hand cleansing and moisturizing creams, mouthwashes, astringents, anti-freckle lotions and beauty masks.

Bran

Bran is the tough outer fibre which covers wheat grains; when the meal is sifted, the valuable bran is left behind. Bran constitutes only 14 per cent of the entire growing wheat grain, but contains comparatively high proportions of protein, riboflavin (vitamin B_2), thiamine (vitamin B_1) and pantothenic acid, all of which are rich when taken either internally or applied to the body. Packets of bran are relatively inexpensive and are stocked by grocers, delicatessens, larger chemists' and health shops.

Bran is still vastly underrated. Those who like to feel that their soap is actually benefiting their complexion rather than just lightly skimming over the surface might like to include bran in one of the gels or soap substitutes described on pages 165–8. The minute and slightly abrasive particles will penetrate deep into the pores and remove specks of dirt, grease and ingrained grime. A facial scrub used with the soap is particularly good for those with extremely greasy complexions, and dead skin collecting on the body should also be regularly massaged away with the help of a body scrub. Your hair will also benefit from an occasional dry bran shampoo for, although it rids the hair and scalp of dust and grime, it does not remove the essential oils as do so many wet detergent shampoos.

Brewer's Yeast

The Ancient Greeks and Romans used brewer's yeast in a variety of cures, but today it is a vastly underrated nutrient. Cheap and rich in essential vitamins, minerals and proteins, brewer's yeast taken internally boosts the circulation and improves the overall condition of the hair, skin, teeth and nails. It has a deep-cleansing action on the skin when applied externally and is frequently incorporated in face masks.

Brewer's yeast, in both tablet and powdered forms, may be obtained from chemists, supermarkets and health shops.

Buttermilk

Buttermilk is the watery residue left over from butter-making and although low in fat it contains roughly the same nutrients, protein and calcium as fresh milk. In Britain, buttermilk is stocked by only some supermarkets but it can be found in the majority of health shops.

It is a deep-cleansing and bleaching agent which is especially helpful for those with oily skins. It can be used in a range of home-made products, including freckle-bleaching creams, large-pore and oily-skin facial cleansing creams, masks, milks and body packs. It is gentle and soothing, and is one of the few natural substances that cool and alleviate sunburn.

Castile Soap

The term 'Castile' was once generally used to describe a white soap without perfume made from olive oil and caustic soda. Today, with so many brands on the market, the name is usually applied to any white and unscented soap made from a variety of popular oils and tallow. By shopping around, you can still find the original article; castile soap is still sold by better chemists' and health shops. The alternative is to buy a selection of relatively inexpensive and small plain bars and do a simple test using a strip of Nitrazine paper (available from chemists). Wet the soaps and place a piece of the paper on each one. The paper that remains yellow (not turning blue, mauve or grey) will indicate which soap is the most acidic and consequently the best for your skin and for making cosmetics and toiletries.

Castile soap may be used in the making of many mild and pleasant natural toiletries, including shampoos, cleansing creams, gels and soaps.

Castor Oil (Ricinus communis)

The Ancient Egyptians used castor oil, and the seeds from which the oil is extracted have been discovered in their tombs. The plant Ricinus communis first reached Greece during the fourth century BC and the plants have been widely cultivated there ever since. Throughout the Middle Ages it was used for medicinal purposes and by the eighteenth century it was common in English gardens.

R. communis may reach a height of around twenty feet (6 metres) in its natural environment but rarely exceeds five feet (1.5 metres) when treated as a tender annual and bedded out in the public parks and gardens of Europe. The large palmate leaves are mid-green to bronze, and remind me of the much smaller Fatsia japonica, a houseplant which is found in many homes.

Castor oil is easily obtainable from chemists', supermarkets and health shops. The oil is used extensively in the commercial manufacture of lipsticks and soaps, and may be included in a number of home-made cosmetics. It is rich and smooth; when incorporated in a conditioning and dandruff-prevention oil, it quickly counteracts harmful drying caused by chemical dyes, Summer sun and salty sea air. It will help to keep the most sophisticated hairstyle beautifully tidy.

Castor oil is excellent for strengthening nails and also provides a fairly varied range of body oils, lip glosses and bath oils, each of which will enrich and benefit the driest of skins.

Cinnamon (Cinnamomum zeylanicum)

Until 1776, Dutch merchants had a complete monopoly of the cinnamon trade, yet this spice was harvested only from self-sown trees which grew quite naturally in the wild. Cinnamon spice comes from neither a fruit nor a nut, as one might suppose, but the inner bark of the cinnamon tree which, when dried, tastes and smells sweet and is highly aromatic. The essential oil that it exudes contains a very powerful antiseptic called phenol, which discourages many forms of bacteria. The bark and oil are occasionally obtainable from the spice counters of craft shops and delicatessens, although they are more likely to be found in herb and health shops.

Both the essential oil and cinnamon sticks may be combined in a variety of highly aromatic and luxurious cosmetic preparations. After a bath or shower, treat yourself to a pampering all-over body rub using the exquisite and skin-softening body oil described on page 169. Cinnamon also makes a skin vinegar that is beneficial if used before going out into the sun. It makes a spicy tooth powder and a splendid breath deodorizer.

Cloves (*Syzygium aromaticum*)

Cloves were used by the Chinese thousands of years ago and, by the beginning of the first century AD, a lucrative trade had been established between the spice islands of the East Indies (now known as the Moluccas) and Europe. By the sixteenth century the Portuguese and later the Dutch had the virtual monopoly of the Spice Islands trade, but despite all their efforts this very valuable and expensive crop began to be cultivated elsewhere. There still exists in some places an ancient superstition that children may be protected from evil spirits by wearing beads of cloves around their necks.

The tall evergreen trees produce pink flower buds, but they are not allowed to bloom. Instead, they are picked and dried in the sun, where they turn a reddish-brown and become the well-known spice which is exported all over the world. Ground and whole cloves are obtainable from chemists and most food shops.

Cloves possess powerful antiseptic qualities and make excellent mouthwashes and breath fresheners. They also make a rejuvenating clove foot-bath. You will smell deliciously spicy and feel thoroughly refreshed after a body-splash with clove cologne.

Coconut (*Cocus nucifera*)

There is an old Chinese legend concerning the coconut which tells of two princes, Lin-yi and Yue. The first prince had a great hatred for Prince Yue and sent an assassin to murder him. The killer successfully completed his mission, cutting off Yue's head, which, the story goes, fell into the branches of a palm tree. There it remained hanging, and was duly transformed into a coconut — which is why these nuts always possess two perfect 'eyes' in their shells.

The coconut palm is a native of Malaysia, although it is now cultivated throughout many of the tropical regions. The shell contains the sweet, drinkable milk, but it is from the dried flesh, known as copra, that the valuable oil is extracted.

Coconut oil is obtainable from larger health food shops and chemists. Blended with other ingredients, the white oil makes a super nourishing pre-wash hair-conditioning cream and also plays an integral part in many special sun-tanning lotions, lip salves, soaps and moisturizing creams for hands and skin.

Corn

Corn has played a prominent part in many of the ancient civilizations, and the Romans, Egyptians, Syrians and Greeks all had their own ritual corn festivals to honour their particular goddesses. The Chinese revered corn as a gift from heaven, and twice a year, before sowing and after harvesting, they offered sacrifices and prayers in thanksgiving. In the tombs of Egyptian pharoahs, archaeologists have found that the mummified remains are often accompanied by caskets containing ears of corn. After several thousand years, many grains proved still to be fertile, actually germinating and sprouting into growth.

Corn meal and corn oil are products obtained from this grain, whilst cornflour is a refined starch extracted from maize or Indian corn. Maize, also known as sweet corn, was originally an American crop and was brought to Europe by Christopher Columbus. Corn meal, oil and cornflour are available from supermarkets, delicatessens and health shops.

Cornflour possesses healing properties and is an obvious ingredient of face masks for alleviating sunburn and acne. The milled meal has been used in facial masks, hand creams and complexion scrubs for centuries, and it is as good today as it has ever been.

I found the 'starch' excellent in dry shampoos. Keep a little of the corn oil — it blends well with all sorts of cosmetic creams and tanning oils.

Dairy Cream

Cream is the oil and more fatty part extracted from milk; its thickness and consistency varies according to the type of cream you buy. For instance, single cream is usually homogenized, and possesses far less buttermilk than does double cream, which often contains not double but treble the quantity in single cream.

Many of us indulge in eating lashings of cream, but I always feel that cream is far more beneficial when applied externally, for it is a very pure source of protein and easily absorbed by the skin. At least once a week I try to massage a generous amount of double cream into my skin during the early part of the evening, keeping it on until bedtime, then rinsing it off, toning and applying one of my favourite night creams.

Cream can also be combined with other high-protein concoctions to make it more nourishing; and some of these mixtures are particularly helpful in erasing laughter lines on the delicate areas around the eyes. It is also perfect in all sorts of facials and masks, and if you find that you have some cream to spare, try working it into your neck with gentle upward strokes of the hand, and massaging into your hands and the soles of your feet.

Eggs

Many people believe that brown eggs are more nutritious than white, but although the brown ones certainly look more appetizing, they both contain the same proportions of protein, iron and vitamins (B_6, B_{12} and D). Most of these nourishing substances are in the yolk.

Eggs are one of the oldest and most valuable ingredients of beauty preparations, and it is wise to keep a ready supply. They will keep for months in a cool cupboard, after they have been 'doctored' all over with a thin coating of cooking oil.

When using eggs as a cosmetic treatment, remember that the whites are astringent and should not be used daily. They are excellent 'binders' of other ingredients — as we know from cooking — and gently stretch the skin, a property that makes them marvellous in face masks, special line-erasing creams and hair-setting lotions. The yolks are rich in protein and make superb moisturizers, especially for those who are plagued with dry and flaking skin.

Whilst both parts of the egg have their own uses, they are employed together in protein hair tonics, conditions, shampoos and hand barrier creams. Not only do eggs feed and enrich the hair follicles but they give freshly washed hair tremendous body and shine.

Glycerine

Glycerine is a by-product of soap-making, produced during the merging of the fixed oils and fats by an alkali. A completely odourless, colourless and transparent liquid, it is a useful bacteriocide softener and lubricant, which attracts and contains vital moisture when used in just the right quantities. Bottles of glycerine are sold in chemists' and health shops.

Commercially, glycerine is used in hair lotions, and skin and hand creams, all of which can be made with your own pure ingredients at home. Other beauty care preparations, such as astringents, fresheners, bleaching creams, hair shampoos, conditions, hand gels, cuticle creams, sunburn and body lotions, liquid soaps and bath oils can all include glycerine.

Grapefruit (Citrus paradisi)

Grapefruit is believed to have developed either directly from a strain known as the pomelo or as an independent hybrid which could have resulted from the natural crossing of the pomelo and the sweet orange. The grapefruit was not recognized as a species until 1830, although by the 1880s it was cultivated commercially in the U.S.A.

The tree upon which the fruit grows is well-branched and has dark-green foliage. During Spring and early Summer, masses of fragrant white flowers appear, and these are followed by the thick-skinned, yellow fruits.

Although not widely used in pure cosmetic preparations, the fruit smells and feels deliciously cool when incorporated in bath colognes and skin lotions. When there is little time in which to freshen up, the lotions are particularly good to smooth on ankles, wrists, hands, neck and forehead; I usually keep a small bottle with me in my handbag. This fruit may also be used in face masks, hair shampoos and cleansing scrubs and milks.

Honey

For those who are interested in health, honey is a fascinating natural substance. Apart from being the most ancient known sweetening substance, honey has always been closely linked with the quest for radiant beauty coupled with longevity. We all know that honey is derived from nectar collected by bees from the blossoms of plants, shrubs and trees. Yet few of us realize what is pre-digested in this wonderful substance. It contains many vital vitamins and minerals, including potassium. And it is potassium that makes it so valuable, because bacteria cannot survive where an exceptionally high level of potassium is present. There are hundreds of different kinds of honey on sale in supermarkets, herb, health and food stores. For both cosmetic and nutritional purposes it is best to buy only the pure brands which, though a little more expensive, are far superior in quality.

Honey applied to the skin soothes, heals, softens and nourishes. It is an effective and often essential ingredient in many soaps, face creams, milks, masks, hand and body lotions.

Lemon (Citrus limon)

In ancient times, Arabs introduced lemons to Spain; by AD 200 lemons were grown in Greece and Italy and their cultivation and popularity spread to other parts of Europe. Lemon essence is produced in Calabria, Sicily and Nice, where the fresh lemon peel is first roughly shredded on a coarse grater, and then distilled. The lemon tree is irregularly branching and has a grey trunk and oval, evergreen leaves. It reaches a height of around eleven feet (3.3 metres). The five-petalled, fragrant white and pink flowers appear during the Spring and early Summer.

Daily bathing is an integral part of any beauty programme, yet when removing all the harmful oil and dirt we inadvertently wash away the skin's natural acid. The removal of this all too often leaves our faces feeling taut, but lemon can restore this necessary acid balance. However, pure lemon juice also has a drying action and should never be used too lavishly on dry or normal complexions. Lemons contain lots of vitamin C and, being astringent, make good facial masks, skin tonics, cleansing creams and lotions, some of which are specially prepared for dry skins. Lemon hair shampoos have always been popular with fair-haired people. Those you make yourself are free from chemicals and animal substances and, when you notice how superior these are to commercial products, you'll probably want to make your own lemon rinse, setting lotion, soap, nail lotion, cologne splash and hand cream as well.

Mace (Myristica fragrans)

Mace was greatly valued by sixth-century Arabs, and in Europe by the 1100s it was one of the most expensive and highly prized of all spices. Both mace and nutmeg are part of the same tree, the mace being the brilliant red, seaweed-like jacket that protects the kernel, that is, the nutmeg. To produce mace, the outer layer is removed, pressed and dried. It turns a familiar yellowish-brown and becomes extremely brittle.

The evergreen tree has brownish-grey bark, and reaches a height of around forty feet (12 metres). The blossoms are followed by small, yellow, seed-bearing fruits. The tree is grown in New Guinea, the Moluccas, the West Indies and throughout the spice islands of South-East Asia. Mace itself is always to be found in supermarkets, herb and health shops.

When combined with other ingredients, mace makes a fine hair tonic. In my family, a formula has been handed down from mother to daughter for generations, and we all have exceptionally thick and healthy hair. When you're trying out this preparation, you may use up any remaining mace by making a good cologne, mouth-wash and breath freshener.

Mayonnaise

Mayonnaise is believed to have been invented by the chef to the Duc de Richelieu, after the Battle of Mahon. There you have the derivation of its name!

When eaten, mayonnaise is pleasant and nourishing, but when used externally it is even better. It contains vitamin A, protein, lecithin and, (in my recipe) cider vinegar, all of which are necessary for any glowing complexion. Made as it is from oil, eggs and vinegar, it is one of the most complete of all skin foods, and will prove a marvellous moisturizer. It may be used either straight from the jar or 'doctored' to make individual and specialized moisturizers, such as the superb night, neck and cleansing creams described in this book. Mayonnaise is also used in facials and provides all the necessary nourishment for a good pre-wash hair conditioner.

There are many different ready-made brands in the shops. Check the labels to ensure that you choose one of the purer ones without harmful additives. Better still, you can make your own mayonnaise in a few minutes!

Melon (Cucumis melo)

The Ancient Egyptians, Greeks and Romans were all familiar with the common melon, known then as musk melon, and by 1629 it was being cultivated extensively throughout France. The cantaloup melon (Cucumis melo cantaloupensis), a variety of musk melon, originated in Persia and the surrounding Caucasian regions, and was introduced to Rome from Armenia during the sixteenth century. The fruit is a tender annual; the male and female flowers are pollinated either naturally or by hand to produce the large rounded and juicy harvest.

Both cantaloups (which are rich in vitamins B and C) and the honeydew melon are less acidic than the majority of fruits and make superb face masks. There is also a delicious melon cleansing cream — wonderfully cooling — and a light moisturizer, both of which are suitable for all skin types.

Milk

Milk is one of the oldest of all natural products. The Aryan tribes of central Asia were the first herdsmen and their favourite drink was a mixture of milk and honey. The Ancient Greeks drank considerable quantities of mare's and goat's milk.

Until the latter part of the eighteenth century, babies were fed only the milk of either the natural mother or a wet nurse, and when doctors suggested that cow's milk should be used instead, many parents were very reluctant to do so, in case their children developed the horns, tail and other characteristics of a cow!

Milk is such a comparatively inexpensive and yet enriching beautifier that one can afford to be lavish! High in protein, calcium and vitamins, milk is absorbed quickly and easily by the skin leaving it soft and glowing with health.

One of nature's naturally purest products, cow's milk may be used to prepare many face creams, nourishing and cleansing milks, face packs, scrubs and bath mixtures.

Mustard

The Romans first introduced mustard into Britain, but neither they nor the Greeks used it in quite the same way as we do today, preferring to crush and sprinkle it directly on to their food. Around and about the year AD 900 the French monks of St Germain des Prés became famous for their cultivation of this herb, and later it was pressed into dry tablets which were manufactered in Dijon, a province which today produces half of all the world's supply.

By the 1600s, Tewkesbury in England was also becoming well-known for mustard, but by the early 1700s, a Mrs Clements of Durham had discovered a way of preparing a much finer and more superior powder. This won the praise and approval of the Royal Family, and consequently the centre at Tewkesbury gave precedence to Durham. At the beginning of the 1800s, there was a young man called Jeremiah Coleman whose name was destined to become synonymous with mustard and, on the site of his original factory in Norwich, the company bearing his name is still in existence.

The yellow English mustard is a finely powdered blend consisting of the milled seeds of both the black *nigra* and the yellow *alba* mustards to which some wheat flour has been added.

English mustard in powder and paste forms is available from grocers, delicatessens, supermarkets, and health food shops.

Mustard foot baths are both soothing and warming, and are particularly good when one is feeling chilled and under the weather. Those who feel in need of a tonic bath before retiring to bed, might well enjoy the one detailed on page 163.

Myrrh (Commiphora molmol and Balsamodendron myrrha)

The ancient kings of Persia usually wore crowns of myrrh wood. In medieval times it was the custom to make an offering on Twelfth Night. In 1762, King George III dedicated to God the three gifts of gold, frankincense and myrrh.

Growing to a height of almost nine feet (3 metres), the myrrh shrub has knarled boughs and tiny trifoliate leaves. When the ducts contained within the bark break down and form cavities, these fill up with liquid. When cut, the bark exudes this yellowish-white substance, which hardens into a reddish-brown gum. Both the tincture and powdered forms are sold in larger chemists' shops.

The resin has powerful preservative and gentle antiseptic qualities, which is why in the East it was often used in mummification. It is a valuable ingredient in tooth powders, mouthwashes, anti-wrinkle creams and skin tonics. The tincture is an accepted treatment for mouth ulcers.

Oats (*Avena sativa*)

The familiar edible oats of today are believed to have developed from the 'wild oat' (*Avena fatua*). Although these grew in Europe from the earliest time, they did not become established in Britain until the Iron Age.

Unlike other nutritious crops, oats were not revered by the Romans, who believed them to be associated with the devil. Magicians and wizards used them in their 'arts', and fortune-tellers wriggled them around in their hands in order to make them form patterns which supposedly predicted future events — rather as today they use tea-leaves! We can assume that this association with evil was forgotten or dismissed, for in Scotland there is an old tradition that oats ensure a happy and fruitful marriage if placed in the pantry of the new bride and groom.

The ears of oat grain are born on stalks four feet (1.2 metres) high, and surrounded by rough, deeply veined, striate foliage. Oats, in all the various ground and processed forms, are available from grocers', supermarkets and health shops.

The grain is rich in protein, potassium, iron, phosphates, magnesium and silicon. It is extremely nourishing to the skin as well as being nutritious when taken internally. In the form of flakes and meal, oats provide an effective and pure beauty treatment for, though fine and gentle, they are sufficiently abrasive to remove the minutest particles of dirt and grime when used as a facial mask, scrub or soap gel. They leave the skin feeling wonderfully soft and completely clean.

As a basis for many deep cleansing masks, hand whiteners and bath soaks, they are generally superb and may be used on the most sensitive complexions.

Olive (*Olea europaea*)

In biblical times olives represented purity, success and happiness, and indeed were so highly regarded that Moses exempted from military service any man who offered to remain behind to cultivate the olive groves. The oil was used in cooking and was burned in all places of worship.

Being a symbol of victory as well, the twigs were used to crown the winners of the Olympic games; any unfortunate Athenian found abusing or harming the trees was dealt with very severely.

The evergreen *Olea europaea* reaches an average height of twenty feet (6 metres) and has a greyish bark. From the small white flowers are produced the very oily, ovoid and dark-mauve fruits. The rich oil is obtainable from delicatessens, supermarkets and health shops.

Olive oil is one of the finest of all nature's oils and absorbs the burning ultra-violet rays of the sun. It makes an excellent screening suntan lotion and helps to treat brittle nails, damaged hair and parched complexions. In later chapters I have included some of the finest cosmetic remedies for these problems, together with recipes for a rich and pure body oil, a soap and a face mask, all specially designed for those with sensitive and ultra-dry skins.

Orange (*Citrus sinensis*)

There are many customs concerning the orange, the most famous being that brides should either wear or carry sprays of orange-blossom on their wedding day. In Crete they go one better, for newly married couples are usually sprayed with fragrant orangeflower water. Oranges were accepted by the Saracens as an emblem of a fruitful and happy marriage, whilst in other parts of the world they are a symbol of both innocence and fertility. In Brighton there exists an ancient custom of playing a Boxing Day game of bowls using oranges.

Originally from China, the orange is cultivated commercially throughout the Mediterranean and sub-tropical countries. The tree has deep-green, ovate foliage and bears small, sweet-smelling, white flowers during the Spring and early Summer. These are followed by the round, thick-skinned fruits.

Both the peeled orange rind (which should never be thrown away) and the juicy fruit (containing vitamins A, B and C, phosphorus and a number of other nutrients) may be used in numerous beautifying preparations. All of them are fun to make and exciting to use. The range is so enormous that this book includes only some of the finest of the orange skin creams, fresheners, cleansing scrubs, facial masks and milks together with a hand lotion, body cologne, hair shampoo and rinse.

Orris (*Iris germanica*)

Dried orris root was extensively used in all types of perfumery in Ancient Greece and Rome. It was first introduced into northern Italy during the Middle Ages. Orris was widely cultivated there, particularly in Florence. By the fifteenth century orris was being used in Europe not simply to perfume linen and clothing but as a dentifrice and talcum powder.

Iris germanica bears large white flowers tinged with lilac, but it is cultivated purely for its roots. Known as orris, they take up to three years to reach maturity; when freshly harvested they have a very bitter taste, which fades when the root is dried.

The golden oil distilled from the dried powdered roots has a heady fragrant smell of violets and is sometimes known as 'otto of orris'. The dried roots are sold in larger chemists', herb and health shops. The oil is better obtained from one of the aromatic oil companies.

There are occasions when we all want to look particularly good yet haven't the time to wash our hair. These are the times when a reliable dry shampoo is a real boon! I make several, all of which contain orris root — and they are particularly good because they leave your hair clean,

66

shiny and manageable. Orris is also valuable as a dentifrice and helps to keep your teeth beautifully white.

Peach (*Prunus persica*)

The peach, as its Latin name indicates, was believed to have been brought from Persia to Europe by the Romans and was nicknamed the 'Persian apple'. However, we now know that the peach is a native of China, where it is a symbol of longevity.

Poor Sicilians suffering from goitre eat peaches during the nights of Ascension Day and the Feast of St John in the belief that if the peach tree from which the fruit has been plucked dies, it will inevitably take their affliction with it. There is a similar country remedy in Italy: people wishing to rid themselves of warts pluck and bury peach leaves in the ground, believing that their warts will disappear as the leaves decompose.

Prunus persica is a hardy, deciduous specimen, now cultivated both as a bush and a tree. Although the fresh fruits are on sale in fruiterers and supermarkets only during part of the year, both the tinned and dried kinds can be purchased all the year round from supermarkets and health shops. Peach oil is available from many of the larger chemists' and health shops.

Peaches always smell delicious and feel luxurious when applied to the skin. They actually do good as well by enriching, moisturizing and lightly toning tired complexions. This book includes several peach masks and you can have lots of fun deciding which one you like best. There's nothing more revitalizing than a peach and honey mask, which will leave your skin feeling soft and silky. Finish off your nightly beauty routine by pampering your face and body with my floral peach cream, milk and all-over oil! They tone, feed and soften the skin.

Rosewater

The distillation of rose petals to produce rosewater almost certainly originated in Ancient Persia, where the earliest emperors filled the streams surrounding their gardens with this fragrant essence. A document in the French national library in Paris tells us that in AD 810 Persia's leading rosewater manufacturing province, Faristan, was compelled to provide an annual tax to the treasury of Baghdad totalling 30,000 bottles of rosewater.

The art of distilling rose petals was introduced into the West by the Arabs during the tenth century; not long afterwards the French started to manufacture rosewater in the province of Avicenna. It is slightly perfumed, clear and colourless and is available from chemists and the beauty counters of many shops.

Being especially mild, rosewater is suitable for all skins and is usually one of the main ingredients of skin-softening creams, astringents and lotions for chapped hands. It helps to make a gently moisturizing cleansing soap, a mouthwash and face lotion, and is also present in perfumed waters, colognes, masks, bath oils and shampoos.

Safflower (Carthamus tinctorius)

The safflower plant was first introduced into Europe from Egypt in 1551. The seeds from which safflower oil is extracted are eaten by the poorer people in some parts of the world, whilst in Poland the flowers are used in the making of bread and other food-stuffs. The flowers also contain an excellent red dyeing agent known as carthamin, which is used to colour silks, linen and cosmetics, and is mixed with French chalk to make rouge.

The safflower plant is a thistle-like annual with white stalks and pointed oval foliage, which reaches an average height of two to three feet (60 to 90cm). The red, orange or yellow flowers are followed by white, four-sided fruits, which when pressed yield the pale yellow, oily liquid. The oil is obtainable from delicatessens, grocers and health shops. It is nourishing and may be included in almost any facial moisturizer, cleanser and body oil. When blended with other ingredients and used regularly as a bath oil, it will leave your body feeling pampered and silky soft.

Salt

Salt has powerful cleansing and healing properties and may be used in an assortment of top-to-toe home treatments. These range from face creams and hair shampoos to dentifrices, mouth washes, handpastes, reducing and rejuvenating bath mixtures, nail oils and foot-baths.

Table and cooking salt (the purer of the two) are obtainable from grocers and supermarkets, whilst sea salt is more likely to be found in delicatessens, chemists' and health shops.

Sesame (Sesamum indicum)

Sesame plants were cultivated in the East thousands of years ago and were used by the ancient and advanced civilizations of Persia, Egypt and Greece. Sesame oil is still used by the inhabitants of many hot countries because, unlike other oils, it does not become rancid in extremely hot weather.

The sesame plant is an erect-growing annual that reaches a height of nearly six feet (1.8 metres). It bears pink-and-white tubular flowers and later oily seeds which, depending on the strain, vary in colour from red to black, brown and white. Both the seeds (which contain sixty per cent oil) and the extracted oil are on sale in supermarkets, herb and health shops. The paste made from the oil, known as tahini, is available in some health shops as well as in Greek shops.

Sesame oil absorbs the sun's often harmful ultra-violet rays, and so is particularly useful when compounded in suntan lotions and other creams which are specially intended for use in summer. There is also a variety of all-purpose skin foods and hand lotions, in which sesame oil plays an important role. Mixed with other ingredients, tahini makes a super-fine toning face-mask.

Sherry

Sherry is made from certain grape juices and the best comes from the areas around Jerez de la Frontera in southern Spain. By the reign of Elizabeth I, sherry was an established drink among the English aristocracy and by the 1700s it had become a popular drink enjoyed by both rich and poor.

Originally, in sherry-making, the grapes were crushed under foot by men wearing specially designed boots, which had nails for piercing the fruit and extracting the juice without releasing the pips. Once the grape juice is extracted it is allowed to ferment, always tended and fed by the winemakers, then held in stock by the various shippers until it has matured.

In this book I have generally avoided those ingredients which are suitable for only one or two recipes — unless they are of special importance. Sherry is one that I really could not exclude, even though I use it in only a single recipe, because it makes a wonderfully spicy mouthwash and breath freshener.

Sour Milk and Sour Cream

Sour cream is consumed throughout Rumania, Germany and Eastern Europe. When talking of 'soured' cream or milk, we are really referring to the somewhat acid flavour which is caused by the presence of lactic acid. Being a preservative, this acid tends to conserve essential vitamins in the milk or cream and as an active substance it also attacks bacteria, dust and grime.

Sour milk, sometimes referred to as 'cultured milk' or 'acidified milk', is occasionally sold by dairies and, like sour cream, is sold in the larger supermarkets and health shops. However, it is easy to keep a little fresh milk outside the refrigerator, and let nature do the rest! If you wish, you can hurry it up by adding a few drops of lemon juice, but I find that the naturally soured variety is better.

I treat my skin every day to an acidified milk and cream facial rub, which is absorbed easily and keeps the complexion looking young, firm and well-nourished. Both the soured milk and cream act as softeners, make efficient skin foods and cleansers and help to eliminate enlarged pores.

Tea (Camellia sinensis)

Tea is generally believed to have been taken in China as early as 2737 BC, but it was not until AD 350 that it was first mentioned in Chinese writings. It was introduced to England in 1661, when Samuel Pepys tasted it for the first time, according to his diary. Two years later, the almost-legendary East India Company presented two pounds of tea to the monarch, Charles II; presumably he liked it, for by 1664, tea was being sold in London for the astronomical figure of £3 a pound.

Camellia sinensis has deep-green elliptical leaves and produces white blooms, which are followed by round, seed-bearing fruits. The so-called tea plant is an evergreen shrub which may reach a height of thirty feet (9 metres) when allowed to grow unchecked; when cultivated it is restricted to a more manageable eight feet (2.4 metres). To produce the familiar beverage, the leaves are gathered, exposed to the air and then tossed, roasted, rolled, sometimes fermented, and pressed several times before they are finally dried.

The tannin in tea has no nutritional value at all but it is widely used in treating skin diseases. Because tannin absorbs the sun's harmful ultra-violet rays, tea is useful as a screening lotion. Tea also aids the tanning process by initially browning wintry-white skins. A tea rinse will highlight dull brown hair and gently colour grey hair. When your eyes are particularly tired, cover them with tea-soaked pads of cotton wool and they will quickly sparkle again.

Tragacanth

Gum tragacanth, also known as Syrian tragacanth, is a gum-like resin exuded from incisions made in the bark of the *Astragalus gummifer* shrub. When cuts are tapped, the tragacanth which first collects is white but as the resin flows more freely it becomes a lemon-yellow colour. It trickles out to form thin, ribbon-shaped 'tears' and in drying it loses approximately 14 per cent of its water content. When solidified, it is quite brittle and is easily collected for commercial use.

The thorny, bush shrub is found growing in Iran, Turkey, Greece and the southern and eastern parts of Europe. The yellowish, powdered tragacanth is both tasteless and odourless and will only partially dissolve in water. However, it is completely soluble in an alkali. It is obtainable from chemists and health shops.

As a thickening emulsifier, tragacanth is used in the manufacture of toothpastes and hair wave preparations. At home it is useful in making hand gels, creams, and non-oily hairdressing lotions. When not in use, tragacanth *must* be stored in a dry place.

Vinegar

Vinegar has been in use for at least five thousand years, possibly longer. The word 'vinegar' is derived from the French *vin aigre* meaning 'sour wine', and vinegar is the eventual product of the fermentation of the juices of almost any kind of fruit or berry.

Vinegars are widely used in the kitchen, but as a beauty aid they have remained vastly underestimated. This is a great pity, for there are few types of preparations in which they cannot play a useful part.

Millions of pounds are spent yearly on chemically produced toiletries to make bathing a more relaxing, luxurious, and pleasurable pastime. But you can make a series of aromatic bath vinegars at a fraction of shop prices. Cider vinegar is particularly good for your body, face and hair, and this vinegar can also be used in hair lotions, anti-dandruff preparations, cleansing and nourishing creams, skin tonics and suntan oils.

Vodka

Vodka is believed to have originated in the Russian fort of Viatka during the twelfth century. There is little doubt that the spirit was then made from potatoes, although it is now produced from grain. The word *vodka*, means 'little water', and is the shortened version of its original longer name, *zhiznennia voda*, meaning 'water of life'.

A pure alcohol of one kind or another is needed in certain types of cosmetic preparations — there is no real substitute. Many mouthwashes, colognes and perfumes have an alcohol base, as indeed do certain hair lotions, dandruff treatments and astringent tonics.

It is quite safe to substitute ethanol or industrial alcohol for vodka in these recipes if you can obtain it.

Wheatgerm

Wheatgerm, not wheat flakes or wheat bran, is the wheat embryo, the spark necessary to give life to new plants, and is contained in the heart of each grain. Wheatgerm constitutes only 3 per cent of the grain, the remainder consisting of bran (14 per cent) and the starchy endosperm (83 per cent). Wheatgerm is removed during the milling process, and is particularly valuable because it contains appreciable quantities of vitamins A, B_1, B_6 and E, as well as copper, magnesium, phosphorus and calcium. It is perishable and once the producer's airtight covering has been removed it can be kept in a screw top jar for only a short while — the quicker it is used, the better! Vacuum-packed wheatgerm is available from many larger chemists', supermarkets and food stores. The wheatgerm oil, in capsule form is on sale in herb and health shops.

Dried wheatgerm, which is an important component of any nutritous eating programme, may also be used in some dry shampoos and face scrubs, masks and creams. The oil extracted from the wheatgerm is generally more easily incorporated in moisturizing and under-eye wrinkle creams. It is very valuable in such products, being rich in phosphorus and many vitamins, including vitamin E. It soothes, heals and helps to feed and smooth out any crêpy lines and wrinkles.

Yogurt

Plain yogurt is a pure milk product containing no artificial additives, which has a sour though not unpleasant taste. A very popular food in many parts of the world, particularly the Balkans, yogurt is a marvellous internal and external beautifier. It is also one of the safest, for the majority of disease-producing organisms are killed off by the acid it contains.

The beneficial effects of yogurt are many and, although it is delicious to eat, always try to leave a carton or two in the refrigerator for external applications as a beautifier. Yogurt is frequently mixed with other pure ingredients to make face masks, scrubs, moisturizers and cleansers, many of which are suited to both combination and oily skins. They are also of special value to those with acne, slight spots or pimples. Try yogurt too as a hair conditioner.

Additional Natural Ingredients

You will find these additional natural substances to be useful beauty aids. Most are easily obtainable and need little description.

Substances	Properties	Uses
Apricot kernel oil	moisturizes and softens	skin tonics and conditioners
Arrowroot	thickening agent	hand creams, dry hair shampoos, toothpastes
Baby oil	cleanses	cleansing creams
Barley	cleanses, soothes, heals	masks
Benzoin	soothes and restores	skin preparations
Bicarbonate of soda	cleanses	dentifrices, mouthwashes, hair shampoos
Brandy	cleanses and preserves	skin tonics, hand lotions, bath oils, hair conditioners
Calamine lotion	soothes	sunburn lotions
Carrot oil	rich in vitamin A	skin preparations
Chillies	stimulates hair growth	hair tonics
Cocoa butter	cleanses, nourishes and softens	suntan oil, lip gloss, cleansing, throat, night and hand creams
Cod-liver oil	rich in vitamins A and D	skin preparations
Fullers' Earth	cleanses, and has good 'drawing' powers	hand barrier creams, dry hair shampoos, masks
Garlic	antiseptic, stimulates hair growth	hair tonics and conditioners
Gelatine	animal protein rich in collagen	skin preparations
Henna	dye and conditioner	hair colourant
Hibiscus flowers	weak dye	hair colourant
Indigo leaves	dye	hair colourant
Iodine	antiseptic, rich in minerals	nail-strengthening lotions, suntan oils

Substances	Properties	Uses
Iron	carries oxygen to the skin	skin preparations
Jojoba oil	moisturizes and softens, excellent for sensitive skin	skin conditioners
Kaolin	binds and has good 'drawing' powers	soap substitutes, hair colouring paste, masks
Lanolin	moisturizes and softens	cleansing, night and throat creams, body and suntan oils, lip salves
Lecithin	rich emulsifying agent	face packs and creams
Liver (desiccated and fresh)	rich in B vitamins, iron and vitamin E	skin preparations
Mineral oil	lubricates and heals	skin preparations
Onions	antiseptic which has good 'drawing' powers	hair lotions and rinses
Peanut butter	nourishes	face and hand creams
Persimmon	nourishes and restores natural acidity	face masks and facials
Petroleum jelly	lubricates and heals	cold creams, lip salves, hand gels, cuticle creams
Rhubarb	dye	hair colourant
Rum	preserves	hair tonics, conditioners, lotions and colourant
Seaweed (kelp)	thickening agent, rich in minerals and collagen-building vitamin C	skin preparations
Soybean oil	polyunsaturated, readily absorbed oil	skin conditioners
Spinach	cleanses. A rich source of vitamin A	masks
Sugar	cleanses and gives body	cleansing creams, hair-setting lotions and hand cleansers
Sulphur	neutralize oiliness and heals	face masks
Surgical spirit	antiseptic	astringents
Tobacco	dye	hair colourant
Turnip	good 'drawing' powers	face masks

Substances	Properties	Uses
Vitamin A	softens, soothes, restores	skin prepations, facials
B vitamins	soothe, nourish	skin preparations
Vitamin C	vital in the formation of collagen	skin conditioners, facials
Vitamin D	heals, lubricates	skin preparations
Vitamin E	heals, smoothes, softens	skin conditioners
Vodka	astringent, cleanses	skin tonics
Walnut	dye	hair colourant
Witch hazel	astringent, soothes	skin fresheners, mouthwash, hand creams

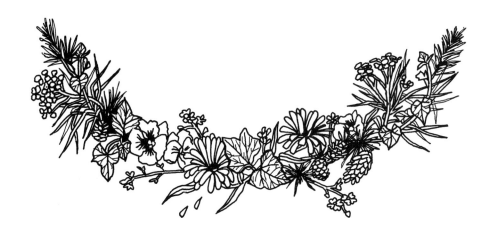

PART TWO

Cosmetics to make at home

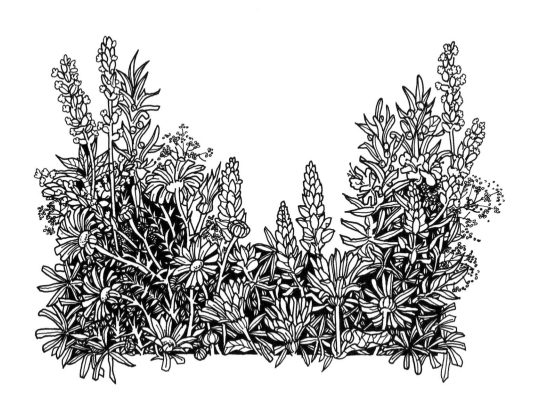

7
For the Face and Eyes

Moisturizing Creams

Floral Fruit Face Cream

Prepare the elderflower water the day before by pouring a pint (570 ml) of boiling water over a good handful of clean, freshly picked blooms. Allow them to steep overnight. Strain.

Place all the oils and wax into a double boiler or a basin suspended over a pan of hot water and stir with a wooden spoon as they slowly melt over a low heat. Remove the pan from the heat and add the elderflower water, in which the borax has previously been dissolved. Add a few drops of perfumed oil (optional) and continue stirring until the liquid thickens and cools. Bottle and label.

3½ tablespoons elderflower water
2 tablespoons olive oil
1½ tablespoons coconut oil
1 tablespoon sesame oil
1 tablespoon almond oil
1½ tablespoons avocado oil
½ tablespoon beeswax
½ teaspoon borax
Perfumed oil (optional)

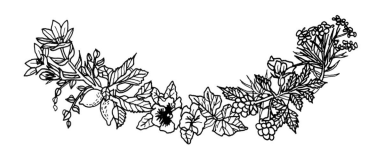

Lanolin and Wheatgerm Night Cream

2 tablespoons
  lanolin
½ tablespoon clear
  honey
½ teaspoon
  glycerine
1 tablespoon
  wheatgerm oil
1½ teaspoons
  lecithin powder
3½ tablespoons soft
  or rain water
Perfumed oil
  (optional)

Place all the ingredients except the water and perfume into a saucepan and, using a whisk, gently mix the contents until they are thoroughly blended. Place the saucepan on a very low heat and gradually add the water. Continue whisking until the mixture looks smooth and creamy; remember that, although it should be warm, it must never become hot. Remove from the heat and add a few drops of your favourite perfumed oil (if desired). When the cream has cooled, bottle it in an airtight jar and label.

The honey, lecithin and wheatgerm contained in this night cream are excellent foods for all skin types. They are easily and quickly absorbed by the skin and help keep it clear, nourished and wrinkle free.

Sesame Honey Cream

20 tablespoons
  sesame oil
3 teaspoons single
  cream
1 egg yolk
1 teaspoon sea salt
1 teaspoon lecithin
  powder
4 tablespoons apple
  cider vinegar
1 teaspoon clear
  honey
Perfumed oil
  (optional)

Blend one-fifth of the sesame oil, the single cream, egg yolk and sea salt thoroughly. Add another four tablespoons of oil and the lecithin and blend again. Add the cider vinegar, honey, and remainder of the oil and a few drops of perfumed oil if desired. Blend the final cream for a further couple of minutes, then bottle and label. It is best kept in the refrigerator.

This nourishing cream is particularly good for those with dry complexions. It is best applied while you are bathing or last thing at night. The beneficial effects are quickly obvious, especially when it is used in conjunction with a light and protective day cream.

Avocado Night Cream

Melt the oil and wax in a double boiler (or similar utensil) over a very low heat. Add the avocado, cream and rosewater. Whisk thoroughly. Dissolve the borax in the water, add to the mixture and continue stirring over a gentle heat for a minute or two. Remove from the heat and keep blending until the liquid cools and becomes smooth and creamy. Pot up and label.

This is a very enriching cream which can be used for all types of complexions, but those with parched or flaky skins will find it invaluable, especially when used in conjunction with a good day cream.

2½ teaspoons avocado oil
1 teaspoon beeswax
1 teaspoon peeled and pulverized avocado
1 teaspoon single cream
½ teaspoon rosewater
1 pinch borax
2 tablespoons soft or rain water

Multi-vitamin Moisturizer for Dry, Tired, or Scaly Skins

Place the mineral, cod-liver and castor oils together with the lecithin in a blender and mix thoroughly.

Dissolve the gelatine in ¼ cup of cold water, then add ¾ cup of boiling water. When cool, add half the gelatinous mixture to the blended ingredients. Whisk in the glycerine, carrot oil, and vitamins B_2 and E. Pot up, label and refrigerate.

This vitamin-packed skin food will nourish and revive dehydrated and lifeless-looking skin.

16 tablespoons mineral oil
½ tablespoon cod-liver oil
½ tablespoon castor oil
2½ tablespoons lecithin
1 tablespoon unflavoured gelatine
1 teaspoon glycerine
1 teaspoon carrot oil
Vitamin B_2 (50mg capsule)
Vitamin E (100iu capsule)

Simple Vitamin Moisturizer

Warm the safflower and wheatgerm oils by placing them in a glass bowl set in a pan of warm water. Add the lanolin and stir continuously until a creamy consistency is reached. Snip off the end of the multivitamin capsule and pour the contents into the bowl. Stir until the pan of water has gone cold. Pot up, label and refrigerate.

2 tablespoons safflower oil
½ teaspoon wheatgerm oil
2 tablespoons lanolin
1 multivitamin capsule

Vitaminized Skin Food for Mature Skins Under Stress

16 tablespoons
mineral water
(fizzy, not still)
1 teaspoon glycerine
1 tablespoon gelatine
1 teaspoon kelp
1 tablespoon vodka
Vitamin B_2 (50mg
capsule)
Vitamin C (100mg
capsule)
Vitamin E (100iu
capsule)

Blend the mineral water and glycerine together. Prepare the gelatine by dissolving it in a ¼ cup of cold water and then adding ¾ cup of boiling water. When cool, pour ½ cup of the gelatinous mixture into the blender along with the remaining ingredients and the contents of the vitamin capsules. Blend thoroughly. Pot up, label and refrigerate.

Skins stressed by anxiety, shock and lack of sleep need the nutritional and toning qualities of this specially-formulated skin food. One can feel the vitamins nurturing the skin. For best results use nightly.

Vitamin Conditioning Night Cream

1 egg yolk
2 teaspoons honey
½ teaspoon
wheatgerm oil
½ teaspoon carrot
oil
½ teaspoon apricot
kernel oil
Vitamin B_2 capsule
(2 drops only)
Vitamin B_6 capsule
(2 drops only)

Beat the egg yolk; add the honey and the wheatgerm, carrot and apricot kernel oils and blend all ingredients. Puncture the vitamin capsules and measure out the required drops. Mix all ingredients together thoroughly. Pot up, label and refrigerate.

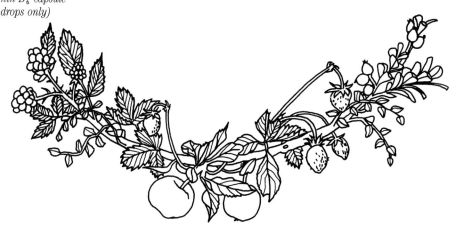

Skin-Preserving Moisturizer with Added Vitamins

Melt the lanolin in a glass bowl set in a pan of boiling water. Remove the pan from the heat and stir in the safflower, apricot kernel and evening primrose oils. Add the lemon juice and beat well. When this mixture has cooled puncture the vitamin capsules and add their contents, stirring all the time. Pot up, label and refrigerate.

This formula helps to preserve, protect and nourish skin that is past its prime. One can feel its regenerative and healing effects.

16 tablespoons lanolin
8 tablespoons safflower oil
2 tablespoons apricot kernel oil
1 tablespoon evening primrose oil
1 teaspoon lemon juice
Vitamin A (10,000iu capsule)
Vitamin D (400iu capsule)
Vitamin E (100iu capsule)

Marigold Moisturizer for Oily Skins

Prepare the marigold water the day before by taking a handful of freshly picked and washed marigold blooms and steeping them overnight in a pint of boiled water. Strain.

Mix in the lecithin and alcohol until smooth, then add the glycerine and the rosewater. Put into a double boiler and stir until the mixture boils. Allow it to simmer on a low heat for about three minutes and then remove from the stove. Continue stirring until the mixture cools.

This moisturizer is particularly good for those with acne or oily complexions because while it feeds the skin the marigold concoction helps to control blemishes and spots. To help eradicate such skin problems this moisturizer is best used in conjunction with an antiseptic cleanser and toning lotion.

2 tablespoons marigold water
1 dessertspoon lecithin powder
2 tablespoons alcohol
1 tablespoon glycerine
1 tablespoon rosewater

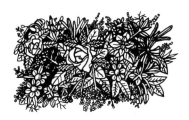

Floral Peach Cream

3 tablespoons peach oil
½ tablespoon olive oil
½ tablespoon wheatgerm oil
1 teaspoon beeswax
1 tablespoon rosewater
1 pinch borax

Melt the wax and oils in a double boiler or similar container over a gentle heat. Dissolve the borax in the rosewater and add. Remove from the heat, and stir continuously with a wooden spoon until the cream has cooled.

To help counteract dryness caused by too much summer sun clean your face thoroughly with a gentle and pure cleansing cream and then a natural soap. Then, generously apply this peach cream over the face and neck. Soaking in a warm bath will encourage the skin to absorb this enriching moisturizer.

Yogurt Night Cream for Oily Complexions

3 tablespoons plain yogurt
1 egg yolk
1 tablespoon single cream
½ tablespoon cider vinegar
½ tablespoon tomato juice
1 tablespoon honey

Mix the yogurt, egg yolk and single cream. Add the cider vinegar and tomato juice. Warm the honey until it becomes runny, add and whisk the mixture until it is smooth and creamy.

Oily complexions vary, some being greasier than others. If after using this recipe three or four times you find the effect is too drying, add a little more cream. If it is not drying enough, add a little more yogurt.

Honey Anti-Wrinkle Night Cream

4 tablespoons milk
2 teaspoons honey
10 tablespoons single cream
1 egg yolk
4 drops tincture of myrrh

Gently heat and whip the milk and honey together. When the honey has dissolved remove saucepan from the heat. Add the single cream, egg yolk and myrrh and whisk vigorously for three minutes. Place in a screw-top jar, label and refrigerate.

This is one of my favourite creams, and I use it daily. At first it may seem slightly sticky because of the honey, but it is quickly absorbed into the skin and once you have used it several times you won't notice the tackiness at all. An excellent anti-wrinkle treatment, it also enhances younger complexions. It is particularly suitable for the most sensitive skins.

Mayonnaise Egg Cream for Wrinkles

Slowly heat the honey until it runs and add to the warm (but not hot) milk. Add the other ingredients and thoroughly whisk the mixture for several minutes. Pour the cream into a screw-top container and refrigerate.

'Tired' complexions that are showing the effects of years of neglect or abuse will derive enormous benefit from this extremely rich treatment. Apply it lavishly to the face and throat, after washing, in the morning and later in the evening. Give it at least an hour in which to be absorbed, before removing any excess with clean cotton wool.

2 tablespoons milk
1 teaspoon clear honey
3 tablespoons mayonnaise
2 tablespoons sour single cream
2 egg yolks
1 tablespoon lecithin powder
1 tablespoon soft or distilled water

Mint Coconut Cream

Prepare the mint infusion in advance by placing three or four sprigs of mint into a tea cup, and fill with boiling water. Infuse it for two hours before straining. Dissolve the borax in the liquid. Place the oils and wax in a double boiler and melt them gently. Remove from the heat and slowly add the reheated mint infusion. Whisk until it is cool.

This fluffy white cream can be used as either a day or night cream and is suitable for dry, normal and combination skins.

4 tablespoons mint infusion
½ teaspoon borax
3 tablespoons coconut oil
2 tablespoons olive oil
1 tablespoon almond oil
½ teaspoon beeswax

Almond Cream for Greasy Complexions

Grate the wax finely, place in a double boiler with the almond oil and heat gently until the wax has melted. Meanwhile dissolve the alum in the warm orangewater and add the solution, drop by drop, to the oil and wax. Add the tincture of benzoin, take the mixture off the stove and whip until it is cool. Beat in the lemon oil and pour into a warm screw-top jar.

My great-grandmother, who was considered something of a beauty, used this cream regularly as a young woman. Even in her eighties she had retained an almost transparent, porcelain-like complexion. Friends with greasy complexions have told me that it is a superb night cream.

4 level tablespoons white wax
4 teaspoons almond oil
1 tablespoon orangeflower water
1 pinch powdered alum
6 drops tincture of benzoin
8 drops lemon oil

Apricot Anti-Wrinkle Skin Food

1 tablespoon lanolin
2 tablespoons apricot oil
1 tablespoon almond oil
1 tablespoon sesame oil
1 tablespoon olive oil
1 tablespoon wheatgerm oil
4 teaspoons lemon juice

Gently warm the lanolin and oils in a double boiler. When runny, add the lemon juice. Remove from the heat and keep whisking the mixture until it is cool.

For the best results from this skin food, your face should first be thoroughly cleansed of all grime and make-up. Tie back your hair and apply the oil generously over your face and neck, not forgetting to pat plenty of it gently underneath your eyes. Like many wrinkle and dry skin treatments it is best used every day and should be given ample time (one or two hours) to enrich dry complexions.

Jojoba Vitamin Cream for Wrinkles and Sensitive Skins

2 tablespoons lanolin
¾ tablespoon jojoba oil
¼ tablespoon apricot kernel oil
¼ tablespoon evening primrose oil
¼ tablespoon cod-liver oil
1 teaspoon freshly squeezed lemon juice
½ teaspoon benzoin
Vitamin E (100iu capsule)

Melt the lanolin in a glass bowl set in a pan of hot water. Add the jojoba, apricot kernel, evening primrose and cod-liver oils and the lemon juice. Blend well, then pour in the benzoin. Beat thoroughly. Finally, puncture the vitamin E capsule, pour in its contents. Blend until smooth. Pot up, label and refrigerate.

Used regularly, this vitamin cream will keep your skin supple and help prevent the signs of further ageing.

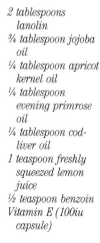

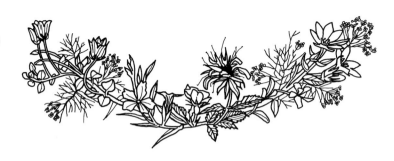

Houseleek Skin Food

Dissolve the borax in the warmed houseleek juice and set aside. Stir the wax, lanolin, almond and wheatgerm oils in a double boiler over a low flame. When they are thoroughly mixed, add the houseleek liquid. Remove from the heat and stir until the mixture is cool. Pot and label.

This recipe combines the healing juices of the houseleek with the valuable vitamin E skin oil (wheatgerm) to make a particularly enriching and soothing skin food.

1 pinch borax
4 tablespoons houseleek juice
4 teaspoons beeswax
2 teaspoons lanolin
1 teaspoon almond oil
8 teaspoons wheatgerm oil

Parsley and Lavender Anti-Acne Skin Food

To make the lavender water, put a handful of lavender blooms into a bowl and pour three pints (1.7 litres) of boiling water over them. Allow to steep for a couple of hours before straining. Bottle the water for future use.

Mix the flour and lavender water to a smooth paste and place it in a double boiler over a low heat. Beat in the oil, and whisk it until it thickens. Remove from the heat, and add the lemon, parsley, salt, myrrh and camomile. Whip the mixture for several minutes, until it has a creamy texture.

A night cream which is excellent for persons with oily complexions inclined to blemishes, spots, and pimples. The best results are obtained when it is coupled with a suitable astringent, cleansing and day cream.

3 tablespoons lavender water
2 tablespoons soya flour
16 tablespoons safflower oil
3 tablespoons finely chopped parsley
½ teaspoon salt
½ teaspoon chopped camomile
10 drops of tincture of myrrh
Juice of ½ lemon

Melon Moisturizing Cream

Melt the oil, wax, lanolin and butter in a double boiler over a low heat. Meanwhile dissolve the borax in the warmed melon juice, and add it to the oils. Remove from the heat, and continue stirring until the mixture thickens and cools. Pot up and label.

You can produce a really big pot of this all-purpose cream, without worrying about how to use it up. The practical thing about it is that, apart from being a rather good moisturizing cream, it also makes a very efficient skin cleanser, and a hand moisturizer as well. So you have three creams for the price of one!

5 teaspoons coconut oil
2 teaspoons beeswax
2 teaspoons lanolin
1 teaspoon butter
1 pinch borax
4 tablespoons melon juice

Multivitamin Skin Food

2 tablespoons white wax
2 tablespoons beeswax
2 tablespoons lanolin
4 tablespoons carrot oil (vitamin A)
4 tablespoons cod-liver oil (vitamins A and D)
4 tablespoons wheatgerm oil (vitamin E)
½ teaspoon ascorbic acid (vitamin C)
1 teaspoon borax
12 tablespoons mineral water
4 drops tincture of benzoin
Vitamin E (100iu capsule)

Melt the white wax and beeswax together in a glass bowl set in a pan of hot water. Add the lanolin, carrot, cod-liver and wheatgerm oils and the ascorbic acid and stir well. In a separate container dissolve the borax in the mineral water. Add the borax solution to the wax and oils mixture and beat until cool. Add the tincture of benzoin and the contents of the vitamin E capsule, and beat until the preparation has set. Pot up, label and refrigerate.

This wonderfully rich skin food penetrates and really nourishes 'starved' and neglected skin.

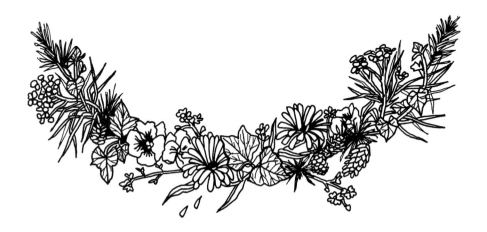

CLEANSING CREAMS

Lavender Cleansing Cream

Melt the wax and the oil together over a low heat. Remove from the heat, and add the lavender water and cider vinegar. Whip vigorously until creamy in texture, and then store in a screw-capped jar.

10 tablespoons
  grated white wax
5½ tablespoons
  almond oil
4 tablespoons
  infused lavender
  water
5 drops cider
  vinegar

Almond and Butter Cleansing Cream

Place the soap and oil in a double boiler, and gently warm them over a low flame until they have melted. Whilst stirring, add the butter and potato water, a little at a time. Remove from the heat, and continue whisking the cream until it cools. Pot up and label.

2 teaspoons finely
  shredded castile
  soap
8 tablespoons
  almond oil
2 teaspoons butter
2 teaspoons strained
  and cooled potato
  water

Cold Cream with Sunflower Oil

Dissolve the borax in the water, and put on one side. Melt the beeswax over a low heat, then stir while adding the sunflower oil. Continue to stir, and meantime, pour in the borax solution. Remove from the heat, and keep stirring while the cream thickens and cools. Pot up and label.

1 teaspoon borax
10 tablespoons soft
  water
5 tablespoons white
  beeswax
18 tablespoons
  sunflower oil

Honeyed Yogurt Cleansing Cream

*16 tablespoons
natural yogurt
5 tablespoons
washed
elderflower heads
2½ tablespoons clear
honey, melted*

Place the yogurt and elderflower heads in a pan on a very low heat and simmer for thirty minutes. Remove from the heat and leave to steep for five hours. Then reheat the mixture, strain and add the melted honey. Whip together for several minutes, bottle, label and refrigerate.

This is a super cleanser suitable for all skin types. Apply generously over face and neck and clean off with a wad of cotton wool. Repeat at least once to remove all traces of make-up and grime.

Mayonnaise Cleansing Cream

*1 egg yolk
1 tablespoon cider
vinegar
½ teaspoon sugar
8 tablespoons olive
oil*

Stir the egg yolk, vinegar and sugar together until well blended. Add the oil, a little at a time. Whip the mixture until it thickens and becomes a smooth, yellow cream. Pot and label.

I knew a woman who after the death of her husband had completely neglected her skin. Although she was only in her mid-fifties, her face was lined and lifeless. I suggested that she should try an intensive treatment using this cleansing cream, mayonnaise egg cream (see page 83) and apricot skin food (see page 84). She did, and within six months looked ten years younger!

Lanolin and Olive Cleansing Cream

*1 tablespoon white
wax
2 tablespoons
lanolin
2 tablespoons olive
oil
2 tablespoons baby
oil*

Place the wax in a double boiler or similar container on a low heat. When it has melted, stir in the lanolin, olive oil and baby oil. Remove from the heat and whip the mixture until it thickens and cools.

Avocado and Lettuce Cleansing Cream

*4 tablespoons lettuce
water
4 tablespoons
shredded beeswax
2 tablespoons
lanolin
7 tablespoons
avocado oil*

First make the lettuce water by infusing three large, clean lettuce leaves in a pint (570ml) of boiling water. Allow to stand for two hours before straining.

Melt the wax and lanolin in a double boiler or similar container over a low heat and add the oil. Stir, remove from the heat and slowly whisk in the lettuce water. Blend until the cream has cooled and pour into a screw-top jar.

Avocado and lettuce cleansing cream feels beautifully creamy and deep-cleanses without leaving any type of skin feeling taut and dried up.

Buttermilk and Lemon Cleanser

Whisk the buttermilk and lemon juice together thoroughly, then store in a screw-top jar. Refrigerate. Apply generously to face and neck and clean off with a wad of cotton wool.

3 tablespoons buttermilk
3 teaspoons freshly squeezed lemon juice

Potato Cleansing Cream

Melt the beeswax over a low heat and stir in the oil. Add the cool potato water in which the borax has been thoroughly dissolved and whisk vigorously. Remove from the heat and continue whisking until the mixture becomes cool and smooth.

This effective cleansing cream also makes a superb hand cream. Because it contains safflower oil and potato water it moisturizes hands while keeping them white and smooth. I often make a double quantity, pour half in a plastic bottle and leave it in the kitchen. Then it's close at hand when I need it.

3¾ tablespoons beeswax
14 tablespoons safflower oil
7½ tablespoons strained potato water
¼ tablespoon borax

Cocoa Butter Cleansing Cream

Place the two margarines in a double boiler or something similar, melt and add the cocoa butter. Stir the ingredients until they are well blended, remove from the heat and whisk until cool.

This is one of the finest cleansing creams I have made and it also serves other useful beautifying purposes. In Winter or Summer, when extremes of temperature often cause the natural oils in your body and hair to dry, cocoa butter cream can be used as a nourishing body cream and pre-shampoo hair conditioner. After you have stepped from a warm bath, apply the cream evenly over your body, concentrating particularly on dry areas such as the undersides of the feet, the knees, elbows and neck.

Used as a conditioner for sun-dried hair, the cream should be massaged well into the scalp and worked down the hair to the tips, where split ends occur. Wrap your hair in a warm towel and leave for two hours before shampooing.

2 tablespoons safflower margarine
2 tablespoons soya margarine
4 tablespoons cocoa butter

Galen's Cold Cream

4 tablespoons olive oil
Highly perfumed rose petals
1 tablespoon purified beeswax
Rain or soft water

Several days in advance place the olive oil in a double boiler and heat slowly until it becomes very warm. Immerse as many rose petals in the olive oil as can be packed in firmly. Cover and leave for several days. When the oil has absorbed the perfume from the petals, strain it and keep on one side until needed.

To make the cold cream, heat the beeswax slowly in a pan until it is reduced to a liquid, then blend in the perfumed oil. Remove from the heat and stir until the mixture cools. Add the soft water, a few drops at a time, until the cream reaches the consistency that you most prefer. Pot and label. Remember thick creams require less water than those with a medium or finer texture.

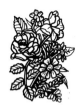

There can be few older cold cream recipes than this in existence, for it was invented by a Greek doctor, Galen, during the second century. It is rich and silky; only after using it, will you appreciate why such a simple cosmetic has survived for nearly 1800 years.

Lavender Cold Cream

11 tablespoons soft water
1 teaspoon borax
5½ tablespoons white beeswax
16½ tablespoons petroleum jelly
16 drops lavender oil

Dissolve the borax in the water and keep on one side. Melt the beeswax and petroleum jelly in a saucepan and add the borax and water solution. Keep stirring the mixture and when cool, add the lavender oil drop by drop, blending all the time. Pot and label.

Cold Cream with Rose Oil

6 tablespoons white beeswax
20½ tablespoons almond oil
6½ tablespoons rosewater
1 teaspoon borax
16 drops rose oil

Place the beeswax in a double boiler and warm slowly until it is runny. Stir in the almond oil. Gently heat the rosewater and borax together in a separate container until the borax has dissolved, then pour the solution into the almond oil and liquid beeswax, stirring all the time. Add the rose oil and continue blending until the cream is completely cool. Pot and label.

ASTRINGENTS, SKIN TONICS AND FRESHENERS

Spicy Astringent Lotion

Mix all the ingredients together and put them in a good-sized preserving jar with an airtight lid. Secure the lid firmly. Keep the jar close at hand to remind you to shake it well several times a day. Leave the contents to infuse and intermingle for seven to eight days. Strain, bottle, shake well and label.

    This makes a zingy and spicy astringent with a fresh unisex perfume.

8 tablespoons alcohol
4 tablespoons rosewater
4 tablespoons orangeflower water
2 tablespoons lemon peel, shredded
1 teaspoon orange peel, shredded
1 teaspoon grapefruit peel, shredded
2 teaspoons nutmeg
2 teaspoons coriander seeds
1 teaspoon cloves
½ teaspoon storax
½ teaspoon benzoin

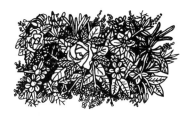

Avocado and Lemon Skin Tonic

Peel and mash the avocados and, when nice and pulpy in consistency, extract the juice by straining it through a square of gauze or a kitchen sieve. Squeeze the lemons and mix the two juices together. Bottle, shake well, and label.

3 over-ripe avocados (large)
1½ lemons (small)

Fruity Skin Tonic for Oily Skins

Peel and mash the cucumber and apple until they are reduced to pulp, and then extract the juice by straining them through a piece of fine gauze. Squeeze the juice from the lemons and orange, and mix all of these liquids together with the rosewater and alcohol. Bottle, shake well, and label.

2 lemons
1 orange
1 apple
½ cucumber
2 tablespoons rosewater
2 tablespoons alcohol

All-Purpose Wild Herb Tonic

2 pints (1.15 litres)
  strained white
  cabbage water
2 tablespoons white
  clover heads
2 tablespoons
  chopped
  blackberry leaves
2 tablespoons slice
  marshmallow root
8 teaspoons brandy

Place the flowers, leaves, and shredded root, in the hot cabbage water, cover, and allow the ingredients to simmer for fifteen minutes. Remove from the heat, and leave them to infuse for one hour. Strain, and add the brandy to the liquid. Bottle, shake well, and label.

This all-purpose tonic combines the anti-acne and skin cleansing properties in the white cabbage and blackberry leaves, the antiseptic brandy, the skin 'lightening' action of the white clover heads, and the 'softening' qualities of the marshmallow root. When mixed together, they provide a good all-round complexion tonic.

Marigold Skin Tonic

8 tablespoons
  marigold petals
1 pint (570ml)
  boiling water

Put the marigold petals into a saucepan and add the boiling water. Cover and leave to infuse for three to four hours. Strain, bottle and label.

Marigolds are very useful beautifiers for they possess healing, cleansing and toning qualities. They are invaluable for treating oily skins that are inclined to develop spots and pustules.

Dampen a clean wad of cotton wool with the tonic and apply to the skin night and morning immediately after washing. Then apply your regular moisturizer.

Floral Astringent Lotion for Dry Skin

8 tablespoons
  rosewater
2 tablespoons
  orangeflower
  water
2 tablespoons extract
  of witch hazel
3 drops of eau de
  cologne

Whisk all the ingredients together. Bottle, shake well and label.

Almond Freshener for Dry Skin

Place the ground almonds and half of the rosewater into a container. Using a pestle or similar utensil, pound and crush them until the liquid becomes white and cloudy like watery milk. Strain the mixture through fine gauze into a second holder. Blend in the remaining rosewater, glycerine, borax and almond essence. Bottle, shake well and label.

4 teaspoons ground almonds
6 tablespoons rosewater
½ tablespoon glycerine
4 teaspoons borax
A few drops of almond essence

Edwardian Skin Freshener for Normal Skins

Dissolve the alum in the hot water and put in a jar containing the mixed rosewater and witch hazel. Blend well and stir in the bergamot essence. Bottle, shake well and label.

A few grains powdered alum
1 teaspoon hot water
4 tablespoons rosewater
4 tablespoons extract of witch hazel
A few drops essence of bergamot

Orange Skin Freshener

Wash, slice and score the peel and place in a saucepan. Add the boiling water, cover and allow to steep for two hours. Strain, bottle and label.

Peel from 3 oranges
3 pints (1.7 litres) boiling water

When used daily, this orange freshener leaves the skin looking toned and enlivened. And because this recipe uses only the peel of oranges, it costs next to nothing to produce!

Rosemary Skin Tonic with Brandy

Put the rosemary into the water, cover and allow to simmer for ten minutes. Remove from the heat and leave to infuse for one hour. Strain and add the brandy to the infusion. Bottle, shake well and label.

3 tablespoons dried rosemary
1 pint (570ml) hot water
4 teaspoons brandy

This stimulating tonic has a delightful aromatic and herby fragrance. It is a super complexion booster and may be used on all types of skin.

Special Strawberry Astringent

8 tablespoons
strawberries
8 tablespoons
brandy
1½ tablespoons
crushed camphor
BP

Mash the strawberries until they are reduced to pulp. Place in a jar and add sufficient brandy just to cover them. Cover the top of the jar with a piece of gauze and leave in a warm room. After about a week squeeze and strain the contents of the jar through the gauze, place the liquid aside for later use.

Now you may eat the macerated strawberries, as they are no longer of cosmetic use; this I feel is one of the perks of the job!

Put more freshly squashed strawberries into the strained brandy, add the powdered camphor and leave to stand for forty-eight hours. Strain the liquid into a bottle and label. This astringent is bracing and delicious, in more ways than one!

The second batch of fruit must under no circumstances be eaten since camphor is inedible. However, this does not mean that it should be wasted. It can be wrapped in a small piece of gauze and used as an astrigent bath rub or, alternatively, added to a favourite fruity face mask.

Herbal Apple Astringent

3 teaspoons chopped
mint
2 tablespoons apple
cider vinegar
½ pint (285ml) soft
water

Place the mint in a jar and add the cider vinegar. Screw on the lid and leave for seven days. Strain and pour the soft water into the liquid. Bottle, shake well and label.

Many will appreciate this astringent because it helps improve and refine coarse-looking complexions plagued by enlarged pores. It tones and imparts colour to previously pasty pallor!

Rosewater Astringent with Alcohol

5 tablespoons
alcohol
1 tablespoon
glycerine
10 tablespoons witch
hazel
17 tablespoons
rosewater

Mix the alcohol with the glycerine, beat well and add the other ingredients. Whisk thoroughly. Bottle and label.

This recipe makes almost one pint (about 500ml) of rosewater astringent, but you can make smaller quantities so long as you use the ingredients in the same proportions. For instance if, instead of using a tablespoon as a measure, you use a teaspoon, you will obtain around one-third (190ml) of a pint. The astringent looks very professional and is certainly purer than many found in shops and beauty parlours!

Fennel Astringent with Alcohol

Pour the water and borax into one container and stir until the powder has completely dissolved. Mix the alcohol and rosewater in another container, then add one liquid to the other. Add a few drops of fennel oil. Bottle, shake well and label.

8 tablespoons soft water
1 teaspoon borax
5 teaspoons alcohol
7 tablespoons rosewater
A few drops of fennel or other herbal oil

Tomato Skin Tonic for Oily Skins

Squeeze the tomato and strain the juice through a piece of fine gauze. Add the glycerine and whip the ingredients together. Bottle, label and refrigerate.

1 over-ripe tomato
1 teaspoon glycerine

A tomato tonic will not keep for long periods, so it is best to make only a small quantity at a time — sufficient for just three or four applications. It is a deep-cleansing and toning tonic and an excellent remedy for blackheads. Use generously and apply daily to the greasy areas.

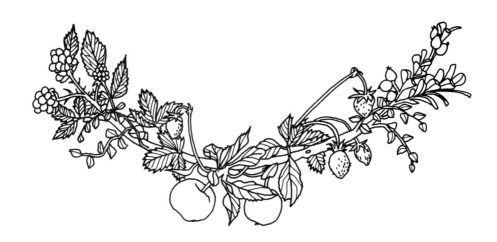

CLEANSING SCRUBS

Orange Yogurt Cleansing Scrub

*1½ tablespoons
natural yogurt
1 tablespoon very
finely shredded
orange peel
1 tablespoon
oatmeal flakes
1 tablespoon
safflower oil*

Stir all the ingredients together until you have an even workable paste. Cleanse off all traces of make-up, before applying the paste to your face, avoiding the delicate areas under the eyes. Using your fingers, massage in small rotary movements for two to three minutes. Rinse with tepid water, and pat dry.

An excellent treatment for blackheads, and being slightly abrasive it rids the skin of deep-seated grease and unwanted dead skin cells. It can be used once a day for those with excessively oily complexions, whilst those with extra dry and normal skins may find it more beneficial to use this orange yogurt cleanser just twice a week, alternating it with the almond meal scrub, which has a slightly less-drying effect.

Almond Meal Cleansing Scrub for Extra Dry Skins

*8 tablespoons
almond meal
3 to 4 tablespoons
melted safflower
margarine*

Add the meal to the melted margarine, and stir until you have a well-mixed and workable paste. If the mixture appears a little too dry for your own requirements, add a little more margarine.

First, cleanse your face of all make-up, then apply the scrub evenly, making sure that you avoid the delicate areas below the eyes. Gently massage in using rotary movements, paying attention to creases around the nose and chin. Massage all over for one to two minutes, before rinsing off with warm and finally cool water. Pat dry. This scrub deep cleanses, tones, and removes all dead cells.

Wheatgerm Cleansing Scrub

*8 tablespoons
wheatgerm flakes
7–8 tablespoons milk*

Warm the milk and add the wheatgerm, stirring until you have a workable paste. Cleanse your face of all make-up and apply the gently abrasive scrub evenly, avoiding the delicate areas under the eyes. Using your fingers, softly massage your skin all over with a circular movement, paying particular attention to the deeper creases in and around the nose and chin. Continue for two or three minutes, before rinsing off with tepid water. Then pat the skin dry.

Such scrubs are very bracing, and they deep-cleanse, tone and remove the unwanted dead top skin, leaving the complexion glowing with health.

Creamed Cornmeal and Grapefruit Cleansing Scrub

Whisk the ingredients together until the mixture is pliable. Cleanse your face of all make-up and spread the paste evenly over your skin. Always avoid the delicate areas below the eyes. Using rotating movements, massage for three to four minutes, paying particular attention to the lines and creases around the nose and chin. Rinse off with tepid water and pat dry.

   This is a superb scrub for those with very dry skins, for while ridding the pores of ingrained dirt it also feeds the skin. Use it as frequently as you wish, even daily.

1 tablespoon fine cornmeal
1 tablespoon grapefruit peel, finely shredded
2 tablespoons soured double cream

Oatmeal and Almond Lemon Cleansing Scrub

Mix all the ingredients together with a fork. Cleanse your face thoroughly, then take some of the mixture in the palm of your hand and mix it with water until you have a soft paste. Spread this evenly over your skin but, as with all the scrubs, take care to avoid the delicate areas below the eyes.

   Massage with small circular movements for two to three minutes. Rinse off with lukewarm water and pat dry.

   This scrub is suitable for all skin types.

1 tablespoon fine oatmeal
1 tablespoon finely ground almonds
1 tablespoon lemon peel, finely shredded

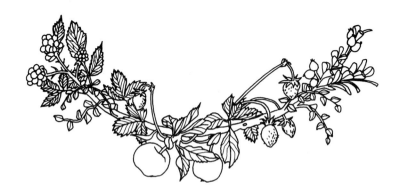

Marigold Bran Cleansing Scrub for Acne

4½ tablespoons marigold water (page 81)
2 tablespoons bran
1 tablespoon sea salt

Add the cooled marigold water to the bran and stir thoroughly. Add the salt and, using a fork, mix until you have a pudding-like paste. If the mixture is too stiff, add a little more marigold water.

Apply the scrub in the usual way and massage your skin for four to five minutes, concentrating particularly on areas prone to spots and pimples, such as the cleft below the mouth, on and around the nose, and the forehead. Rinse with tepid and then cool water and pat dry.

This scrub has an antiseptic deep-cleansing action; it removes dead skin and helps to keep the complexion blemish-free. No external treatment, however good, will completely cure blemishes if you are consuming all the wrong foods. So avoid greasy and very sweet foods and eat lots of fruit and vegetables. Take plenty of exercise in the fresh air, and wash your hair regularly every seven to ten days.

Honeyed Lecithin Cleansing Scrub

1 teaspoon clear honey
2½ tablespoons milk
1 tablespoon lecithin powder
1½ tablespoons kitchen salt

Melt the honey and add the warm milk. Whisk until well blended. Remove from the heat and continue stirring until cool. Then add the lecithin and salt. Blend together with a fork to make a firm paste. Apply the scrub in the usual way and gently massage the skin for three to four minutes. Rinse off with tepid water and pat dry.

This preparation cleanses the skin's surface, penetrates deep into the pores, moisturizes and softens. It may be used on all types of skin.

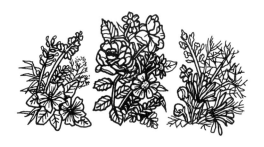

ANTI-FRECKLE LOTIONS AND PASTES

These preparations, because of their bleaching properties, all have extremely drying effects on the skin. Daily treatments, therefore, should never last longer than fifteen to twenty minutes, depending on the severity of the freckles and the individual's skin type. I advocate short treatments daily.

Wash in lukewarm soft water after each treatment, freshen with a suitably mild astringent and nourish with a moisturizing skin food.

Horseradish Lemon Lotion

Steep the horseradish in the lemon juice, and allow it to infuse for forty-eight hours, in a warm room. Bottle, and apply to the freckles, using a wad of cotton wool.

1 teaspoon grated horseradish
Juice of 2 (small) lemons

Dandelion Anti-Freckle Oil

Wash and chop the leaves and place them with the oil in a small pan over a low heat. Allow to simmer for ten minutes, then remove from the heat. Cover and leave to steep for three hours. Strain, bottle and label. This excellent dandelion oil will bleach and fade away stubborn freckles, brown age spots and small moles.

4 medium-sized juicy dandelion leaves
5 tablespoons castor oil

Buttermilk and Oatmeal Paste

Mix the ingredients into a paste. If at first it is too thick, add a little more buttermilk until the paste is easily spreadable.

Spread the paste evenly over the freckled areas and leave for twenty minutes. Rinse with warm water or remove with a suitable light cleansing or astringent lotion.

4 tablespoons buttermilk
2 tablespoons oatmeal flakes

Elderflower and Parsley Lotion

Wash the elderflower blooms and parsley and place in a clean bowl. Cover with half a pint of boiling water and allow to infuse for three to four hours. Strain, bottle, label and refrigerate. Apply to the freckles with cotton wool.

Handful of elderflower blossoms
3–4 sprigs parsley
½ pint (285ml) soft water

Elderflower Cider Lotion

8 tablespoons
   elderflower water
1 tablespoon cider
   vinegar
1 teaspoon alum

Make the elderflower water as in the recipe above, but omitting the parsley. When the elderflower water is cool, add the alum and cider vinegar. Shake the mixture until it is well blended, bottle, label and refrigerate. Apply to freckles using a clean wad of cotton wool.

Lemon Borax Paste

Juice of 1 large
   lemon
1 teaspoon powdered
   borax
1 teaspoon salt

Mix the ingredients into a medium-textured paste, adding more lemon juice if the mixture appears too dry. Spread the paste evenly over the freckles and leave for fifteen minutes. Remove with either warm water or a gentle cleansing lotion.

In addition to the recipes given above, there are several simple treatments that help to bleach freckles. These include infusions of dock leaves, horseradish, lemon balm, lime (linden flowers) and rosemary. Prepare by infusing five tablespoons of leaves or flowers in two and a half pints (1.5 litres) of boiling water for several hours.

Try also the pure juices of cucumber, strawberry or tomato. Other remedies are buttermilk, or a mixture of equal parts of lemon juice and rosewater.

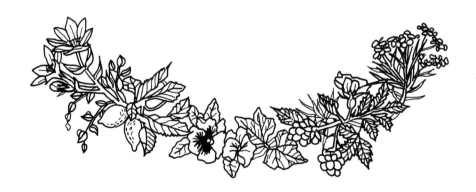

LIGHT CLEANSING/ MOISTURIZING MILKS

These milks are marvellous for removing dust from an otherwise clean and unpainted complexion. They provide the skin with a delicate film which protects against blackheads, prevents excessive dryness and acts as a smooth foundation for cosmetics.

I would never be without them, even though they are no substitute for deep-cleansing and rich moisturizing creams, both of which are vital to the care of all types of skin.

Citrus Milk

Add the lemon juice and the grated peel to the milk, and bottle, label, and refrigerate. Shake it vigorously several times a day, or as often as possible. After twenty-four hours it will be ready for use. It may be strained beforehand, but this is purely optional. Shake well before use.

Juice of ¼ lemon
2 teaspoons grated orange peel
2 teaspoons grated grapefruit peel
¼ pint (140ml) milk

Citrus milk makes a super light, cleansing and toning moisturizer suitable for applying under make-up, as a night milk, or as an all-over body lotion. Applied lavishly, and used regularly, it will keep your skin ultra-silky.

Dandelion and Camomile Milk

Pour the boiling water over the camomile flowers and dandelion leaves, stir well and allow to steep for twelve hours. Add the milk, whisk thoroughly and leave for a further two hours. Strain, bottle, label and refrigerate.

¼ pint (140ml) boiling water
3 tablespoons chopped camomile flowers
2 tablespoons chopped dandelion leaves
¼ pint (140ml) milk

Dandelion and camomile milk is a cleansing moisturizer that is particularly good for rough, sallow complexions. It may be used frequently, but those with extremely dry and parched skins should use it in conjunction with an extra-rich night cream.

Recently, I was introduced to a handsome Romany lady who, though well into her sixties, still possessed a porcelain-like complexion. This, she told me, was largely due to this milk, which she applied daily to her face, neck and hands.

Potato Milk

Boil some potatoes, drain, and strain off sufficient water into a separate container. When cool, add it to the milk and whisk. Bottle, label and refrigerate. Always shake well before use.

4 tablespoons pure potato water
¼ pint (140ml) milk

Strawberry Milk

3 large strawberries, well washed
¼ pint (140ml) milk

Mash the strawberries with a fork, or better still, liquidize them, until they are reduced to a fine, liquid pulp. Add the milk and whisk thoroughly. Bottle, label and refrigerate. Shake well before use.

Strawberries make extremely useful beauty aids because they cleanse and improve the skin's tone and texture. So too does this simple and delicious-smelling milk. And it's good enough to eat!

Almond Milk

½ pint (285ml) milk
4 tablespoons ground almonds

Add the milk to the almonds, and whisk thoroughly. During the next eight hours, stir the mixture frequently, then strain, bottle, label and refrigerate.

This old-fashioned and gentle beautifier makes a superb cleansing moisturizer for dry complexions and may also be used as a daily neck, hand and body lotion.

Note: When you strain the almonds, don't throw them away, for they can be put to further use in a cleansing almond scrub.

Cucumber Milk

2-inch (5cm) piece of cucumber
¼ pint (140ml) milk

Peel, squeeze and mash the cucumber. Place the peel, juice and pulp in the milk. Shake well for several minutes and allow to steep for three hours. Strain, bottle, label and refrigerate.

Mint and Parsley Milk

½ pint (285ml) milk
3 tablespoons mint, freshly chopped
3 tablespoons parsley, freshly chopped

Pour the milk over the mint and parsley, stir well and allow to steep for twelve hours. Strain, bottle, label and refrigerate.

Mint has powerful healing properties and parsley is excellent for controlling excessive oiliness of the skin. Together they make a perfect milk for those whose skins are very oily and prone to blemishes and eruptions. Such skin types still need to be nourished and light antiseptic moisturizers such as this are preferable to heavy and often greasy creams. Mint and parsley milk may be applied to the face both before and after washing in the morning and last thing at night. It is also worth adding a tablespoonful or two to your washing water.

Peach Milk

Add the milk to the peach slices and allow to steep for eight hours. Then strain, bottle, label and refrigerate.

Fresh peaches are unfortunately only available for part of the year. To enjoy the benefits of this delicious, cleansing moisturizer for as long as possible, I make it the moment these fruits come into season, and use it lavishly.

Having made the milk, I usually lie back and massage the strained peach slices into my face and neck for about ten minutes, before rinsing with tepid water. Alternatively, the peach pulp may be mixed with other ingredients to make a face mask. I have always felt that the peach and honey mask (page 106) is the ultimate beauty luxury.

¼ pint (140ml) milk
2 tablespoons fresh peach, skinned and sliced

Extra-Rich Honey Milk

Pour the water into the honey and gently warm until the honey has melted, stirring all the time. Remove from the heat and add the milk and egg yolk. Whisk until well blended. Bottle, label and refrigerate.

I adore using this milk, for it contains some of the purest and richest of all nature's beautifiers. Combined they make a pale yellow milk which cleanses, soothes, softens and enriches the complexion. It makes the skin feel pampered and is good for all skin types and all ages.

2–3 teaspoons water
1 teaspoon clear honey
¼ pint (140ml) milk
1 egg yolk

Carrot and Lettuce Milk

Pour the boiling water over the lettuce and carrot, cover and allow to infuse for eight hours. Add the milk, whisk thoroughly and leave for a further two hours. Strain, bottle, label and refrigerate.

This milk is excellent for all skin types, but because of its cleansing, soothing and healing qualities it is especially helpful for those with sore and very sensitive complexions.

3 tablespoons lettuce leaves, finely chopped
3 tablespoons carrot, grated
7 tablespoons boiling water
14 tablespoons milk

You may also like to try the following simple light cleansing lotions:

Name	To make
Cowslip infusion Elderflower infusion Lemon balm infusion Lime (linden) flower infusion	1 handful to 2 pints (1.15 litres) of boiling water
Plum infusion	3 skinned and sliced plums to 1 pint (570ml) boiling water
Potato water	Cook some potatoes, strain off the water through fine gauze and bottle when cool
Yarrow leaf and flower infusion	1 handful to 2 pints (1.15 litres) boiling water

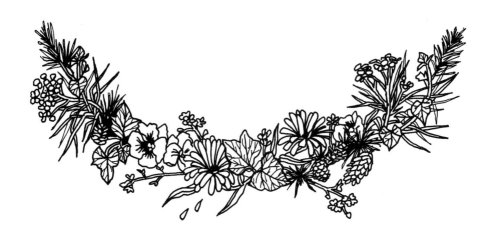

MASKS AND PACKS

Brewer's Yeast Mask for Dry Skins

Cleanse your face thoroughly and either tie your hair back or cover it with a bath cap, so that it is well off your face.

Whisk the first five ingredients together until smooth and well blended. Spread olive or sesame oil evenly over your face, then apply the mask. This pre-mask treatment is most important. Avoid the skin around your eyes. Lie back and relax for twenty minutes.

Remove the mask by splashing your face with a mixture of one part of milk to two parts of soft water. Pat dry, tone and moisturize.

This mask is especially good for dehydrated and tired complexions, for the yeast stimulates the circulation. When used once a week it helps to prevent wrinkles.

1 teaspoon brewer's yeast flakes
2 egg yolks
2 tablespoons clear honey
2 tablesoons sour cream
½ teaspoon cider vinegar
2 tablespoons sesame or olive oil
Milk and water

Protein Cleansing Mask for Dry Skins

Cleanse your face and neck thoroughly and draw your hair well back.

Whisk all the ingredients together into a smooth paste. Apply the mask, using small, circular movements of your fingertips to work it gently and evenly over your face. Avoid the delicate area around the eyes. Pay particular attention to the forehead, the nose and the chin, where blackheads appear most often. Lie back and relax for twenty minutes.

Remove the mash by splashing with clean, cool water. Pat dry, tone and moisturize.

16 tablespoons fine oatmeal
16 tablespoons semi-skimmed milk
½ teaspoon carrot oil
½ teaspoon evening primrose oil
1 egg yolk

Honey Mask with Protein and Vitamins for Dry Skin

Cleanse your face and neck and tie back your hair.

Beat the first four ingredients together, add the contents of the vitamin E capsule and continue beating until well blended. Apply the mask evenly over the face, avoiding the skin around the eyes. Lie back and relax for between fifteen and thirty minutes.

Rinse off with cool water, pat dry, tone and moisturize.

1 egg yolk
1 teaspoon honey
1 teaspoon soybean oil
½ teaspon cod-liver oil
Vitamin E (100iu capsule)

Anita's Bracing Barley Mask

2 tablespoons
   barley, powdered
2 teaspoons mint,
   finely chopped
2 tablespoons clear
   honey
2-3 tablespoons milk

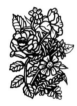

Cleanse your face and neck thoroughly and pin your hair back so that it is well out of the way.

Using a fork, blend the barley, mint and honey together. Add sufficient milk to make the paste smooth and easy to apply without being runny. Apply this invigorating mask over your face and neck, avoiding the delicate area around the eyes. Lie back and relax for thirty minutes.

Remove the mask by splashing with clean, cool water. Pat dry, tone and moisturize.

When I'm feeling overwrought, overtired and overworked, and my skin needs a boost, I treat myself to this food mask. It deep-cleanses, smoothes out tell-tale wrinkles and stimulates the circulation, leaving the skin remarkably silky and supple. In fact, it's just the tonic for any tired-looking skin in need of a pick-me-up!

Peach and Honey Lecithin Mask

½ large peach,
   skinned
3 teaspoons honey
Lecithin powder

Cleanse your face and neck thoroughly and tie your hair well away from the face.

Mash the peach and honey together, add a little lecithin power (half teaspoon at a time) and continue mixing until you have an easily workable paste. Pat this evenly over your face and neck and around the eyes. Don't pull or drag the skin — you will do far more harm than good. Lie back and relax for twenty minutes. Rinse off with tepid water, pat dry, tone and moisturize.

This delicious mask leaves the complexion feeling soft and supple and acts as a real tonic when you are feeling in the doldrums!

Oatmeal Pack for Normal and Dry Skins

2 tablespoons
   oatmeal
1 pint (570ml) water
2-3 tablespoons 'top
   of the milk'
Milk and water

Cook the oatmeal in the water. Cleanse your face and neck thoroughly and tie your hair away from your face.

Strain the cooked oatmeal into a separate container, placing the liquid aside for later use. Mix the oatmeal and 'top of the milk' to a smooth, workable paste and spread it evenly over your face and neck without pulling or dragging the skin. Avoid the sensitive skin below the eyes. Lie back and relax for twenty-five minutes. Rinse off first with the strained oatmeal water and then with a mixture of one part milk to two parts water. Pat dry, tone and moisturize.

This face pack is suitable for the more sensitive skins, being particularly gentle. It both nourishes and heals, and is an ancient and superb deep-cleansing aid.

Spinach Mask for Flaky Skins

Cleanse your face and neck and draw your hair well back from your face.

Wash the leaves and cook them in the milk for about three minutes, or until the leaves are just cooked and still whole. Strain any excess liquid into a separate container and place it to one side for later use. When the leaves have cooled sufficiently to be just comfortably warm, press them flat separately and mould them to the contours of your face and neck. Lie back and relax for thirty minutes. Peel off the leaves and rinse your skin with the spinach milk. Pat dry and tone. Moisturize with lashings of double cream.

8 or 9 whole medium-sized spinach leaves
½ pint (285ml) milk
Double cream

Sulphur Pack for Acne Rashes

Cleanse your face and neck thoroughly and tie your hair back.

Add the epsom salts, sulphur, and starch to the boiling water. Stir well. Whilst still warm, apply the liquid mixture evenly over the affected areas, but keep it well away from your eyes. Lie back and relax for fifteen to twenty minutes.

With clean fingers, peel away the fine crumbly mask. Apply a suitable astringent and light antiseptic moisturizing lotion. The sulphur pack may need to be used only once a week for mild forms of acne; the more severe cases may be treated either once a day or every alternate day.

1 tablespoon epsom salts
1 dessertspoon flowers of sulphur
1 teaspoon powdered starch
16 tablespoons boiling water

Yogurt Clay Packs for Oily and Acne Skins

12 teaspoons fullers'
  earth
2 teaspoons natural
  yogurt
2 teaspoons potato
  water (page 104)

Cleanse your face and neck in the usual way and draw your hair away from your face.

Blend the fullers' earth, yogurt and potato water into a smooth paste. Apply the mixture to your face avoiding the eye areas. Lie back and relax for fifteen to twenty minutes. Rinse off the pack with the remaining potato water, pat dry, tone with an antiseptic astringent and moisturize with a suitable skin food.

Mild acne or a generally oily complexion will benefit from a weekly treatment of this deep-cleansing clay pack. Part of its effectiveness is its drying effect on the skin, so it should never be used more than twice a week.

Vitamin and Mineral Pack for Oily Skins

1 tablespoon
  unflavoured
  gelatine
8 tablespoons
  soybean oil
2 tablespoons sesame
  oil
1 tablespoon
  wheatgerm oil
1 tablespoon cod-
  liver oil
2 tablespoons
  lecithin
2 tablets desiccated
  liver
1 iron tablet
1 vitamin B-complex
  tablet
1 vitamin B_{12}
  capsule

Cleanse your face and throat and pin back your hair.

Dissolve the gelatine in ¼ cup of cold water before adding ¾ cup of boiling water. Stir and leave to cool. Mix ½ cup of the gelatinious mixture and all the other ingredients, including the contents of the vitamin capsule, in a blender. Blend thoroughly.

Apply this mixture to your face and leave for ten minutes. Rinse off with lots of cool water. Pat dry.

The B vitamins in this face pack are helpful in correcting an excessively oily skin.

Fruit Revitalizing Mask

Cleanse your face and throat and tie your hair back well away from your face.

½ ripe avocado, skinned
1 tablespoon fresh tomato juice
1 tablespoon lemon juice

Mash the avocado and add the tomato and lemon juices. Using a fork or potato masher, mix thoroughly. Spread the paste over your face and neck, avoiding the areas around the eyes. Lie back and relax for fifteen to twenty minutes. Rinse off with tepid water, pat dry, tone and moisturize.

In my local fruiterer's there works a woman in her mid-sixties, with a real peaches-and-cream complexion. I naturally assumed that this was due to the large quantities of fruit which she consumes, but she confided that this was almost entirely due to the face creams and masks that she makes from the over-ripe and unsaleable avocados! Women native to very hot countries, the Mexicans for instance, realize the significance of avocados and apply the pulp and rub the oily skin directly on to their faces. This unsophisticated treatment prevents the complexion drying prematurely.

Persimmon Dry Skin Facial

Scoop out some of the pulp from a ripened persimmon, mash it and then add the olive oil, mixing until it is well blended.

1 dessertspoon persimmon pulp
1 dessertspoon olive oil

Cleanse your face in the normal way, and apply the mixture to your face and neck, avoiding the skin immediately below the eyes. Lie back and relax for thirty minutes. Remove with a suitable cleansing milk. Tone and moisturize as usual.

Persimmons nourish and restore the natural acidity often lacking in dry skin. Rich in vitamins A, B_1, B_2 and C, they really work wonders. This fruit only arrived in Britain at the end of 1980, but in America it is a fairly well-known fruit which is both eaten and added to many natural cosmetics.

Hungarian Vegetable Mask

*1 small carrot,
cooked
1 small turnip,
cooked*

Cleanse your face and neck with cleansing cream and tie your hair back well clear of your face.

Mash the carrot and turnip together until well mixed. When cool, spread the paste over your face and neck, avoiding the skin immediately below the eyes. Relax and leave on for thirty minutes. Wash off with a cooling infusion of either lettuce or cucumber and moisturize.

A friend of mine heard of this vegetable mask whilst visiting Hungary. High in vitamins, it gives the skin a gorgeous glow! I only use it once a week, but it may be applied much more frequently and it is suitable for all types of skins.

Orange Honey Facial

*3 tablespoons clear
honey
Juice of ½ orange*

Cleanse your face thoroughly and pin back your hair.

Put the honey and orange juice in a double boiler or similar pan and place over a low heat until it is warm and fluid. Apply the sweet smelling mixture all over your face and throat, including the areas under and around the eyes. It is especially important that the skin surrounding the eyes is never pulled, stretched or rubbed, so the mask should always be patted on. Relax for twenty minutes and then remove the mask with cotton wool and tepid water.

This orange facial is so refreshing that it is a joy to be able to use it all the year round. It is suitable for all ages and skin types.

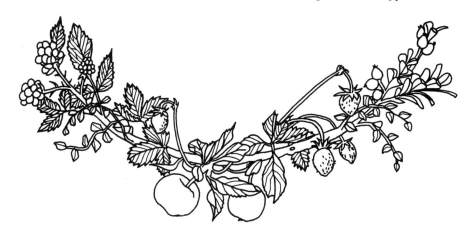

More facials, face masks and packs can be made using the following substances.

Ingredients	Comments
Brewer's yeast, carrot juice and double cream	deep cleanses and nourishes
Cucumber and egg white	for oily skin
Banana and honey	for spotty skin
Banana, carrot juice and lecithin	nourishes
Melon pulp, honey, egg white and brandy	for oily skin
Parsley and yogurt	for oily skin
Blackberry and honey	for eczema
Mayonnaise, sour cream and linseed oil	for dry skin. Very rich and nourishing
Tomato, grapefruit juice and egg white	for oily skin
Tahini (sesame paste) and lime juice	nourishes
Almond meal and milk	for dry, problem skin
Almond meal, mayonnaise and banana	for very dry skin
Plum and brewer's yeast	deep-cleanses
Lime juice, milk and brandy	facial for oily skin
Fennel juice (or infusion), yogurt and kaolin	deep-cleanses
Dandelion soaked in honey	for spotty skin
Wheatgerm flakes (or flour) and sour cream	nourishes
Buttermilk, egg white and lime juice	for oily, sallow skin
Papaya, banana and butter	peels off dry, coarse skin. Leave on the skin for only 5 minutes
Oatmeal and peach	cleanses and nourishes
Melon pulp, yogurt and kaolin	cleanses and refreshes
Apple pulp, oatmeal and witch hazel	tones and cleanses
Peach, honey and mayonnaise	nourishes and softens tired-looking skin
Olive and apricot oils	enriches, nourishes and heals

These treatments should be allowed to remain for fifteen to thirty minutes, depending on your skin type.

Eye tonics, lotions and packs

Herb	To make	How to use
Camomile	Infuse a handful in 1 pint (570ml) boiling water	compress
Cornflower	Infuse a handful in ½ pint (285ml) boiling water	compress
Elderflower	Infuse a handful in 1 pint (570ml) boiling water	compress
Eyebright (dried)	Infuse 1 dessertspoonful in 1 pint (570ml) boiling water	compress
Golden seal	Infuse a handful in 1 pint (570ml) boiling water	compress
Marshmallow	Infuse a handful in 1 pint (570ml) boiling water	compress
Lotions		
Fresh apple juice		eyebath
Fresh carrot juice		eyebath
Packs		
Cucumber		place a slice over each eye
Groundsel (mash well)		place a small quantity on each eye
Teabags		place a cold bag over each eye

Flour Face Pack

2 tablespoons flour
2 tablespoons clear honey
2–3 tablespoons milk

Cleanse your face and neck thoroughly and secure your hair well away from your face.

Whisk the flour and honey with sufficient milk to make a smooth paste. Apply the mixture over your face and neck, keeping well clear of the sensitive skin around the eyes. Lie back and relax for thirty minutes. Remove with lashings of tepid water, pat dry, tone and moisturize.

This simply beauty mask has been known for several hundred years and is still quite popular. Ideal for all types of skin, it is superb for refining and softening complexions that have been roughened by long periods in the hot sun. When used regularly and in conjunction with rich skin foods, it also helps to discourage premature wrinkles and ageing lines.

Honey Refining Mask

Cleanse your face and neck several times using a deep cleansing cream. Tie back your hair or wrap in a towel or bathcap.

2 tablespoons clear honey
1 tablespoon almond oil

Mix the ingredients together thoroughly on a saucer and, with your finger tips, apply the refining mask over your face and neck, avoiding the delicate skin under the eyes. Gently massage the mixture into the skin using circular movements for three minutes. Lie back and relax for a further twenty-five minutes or so. To remove the mask, splash with lashings of clean, tepid water. Pat dry, apply a mild astringent and moisturize.

This honey treatment removes dead cells and the impurities below the surface of the skin. Women of all ages will benefit from a weekly treatment, and it will prove particularly helpful for those with enlarged pores, acne, and dry, rough or coarse skins.

Avocado Egg Mask

Cleanse your face and throat and pin your hair well back from your face.

1 ripe avocado, skinned
1 egg white
1 teaspoon lemon juice
Milk and water

Using a potato masher or fork, blend the ingredients together until you have a smooth and workable mixture. Apply the mask over the face and neck, avoiding the skin immediately surrounding the eyes. Lie back and relax for fifteen to twenty minutes. Rinse with a mixture of one part milk to two parts soft water. Pat dry, tone and moisturize.

Skins of all ages and all types will reap the rewards of this mask, but those of you with dry or normal complexions could of course, apply a much richer night cream than those with oily or combination skins.

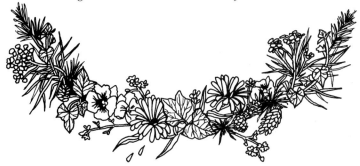

8

For the Mouth and Lips

TOOTHPASTES AND POWDERS

Sage Stain-removing Powder

2 tablespoons fresh
  sage leaves
2 tablespoons sea
  salt

Put the ingredients in a bowl and, using a pestle or some other heavy, smooth tool, crush them into a fine powder. Place the mixture in a warm oven. When it is well baked and fairly hard, remove and pulverize a second time. Store in a shallow airtight container.

This sage cleanser rids the teeth of harmful plaque and unsightly stains and will leave the mouth and breath smelling fresh and sweet.

Almond Toothpaste

2 tablespoons
  almonds, finely
  ground
2 teaspoons
  camphor BP
1 level teaspoon salt
Soft water
A few drops of any
  flavouring
  essence

Place the camphor, salt and almonds into a bowl. Use a pestle or similar tool to pulverize them into a powderlike consistency, mixing them all the time. Add sufficient soft water to make a smooth paste. Stir in the flavouring essence. Store in a small screw-top pot and label.

Cinnamon Tooth Powder or Paste

Mix the ingredients together, pot and label.

    If you prefer to use a paste rather than a powder, add to the above ingredients just sufficient witch hazel to produce a smooth, stiff paste.

8 tablespoons powdered arrowroot
4 tablespoons ground cinnamon

Goldenseal Tooth Powder or Paste

Stir the ingredients together and pot in an airtight container.

    This antiseptic powder may be added to water to make a super mouthwash or paste.

4 tablespoons powdered goldenseal
4 tablespoons powdered gum myrrh

Orris Root Tooth Powder

Mix the ingredients together and pot in an airtight jar.

15 tablespoons baking powder
1 tablespoon orris root

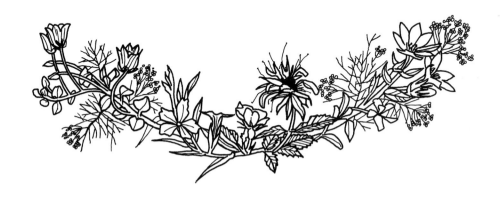

MOUTHWASHES

Simple Mouthwash and Gum-Strengthening Powder

3 tablespoons baking
  powder
3 tablespoons
  kitchen salt

Mix the ingredients and pot in a screw-top jar. To use, stir one teaspoonful of the powder into half a tumbler of water for an instant mouthwash.

Regular daily use will ensure that the breath remains sweet. It also helps strengthen weak, spongy gums.

Quince Mouthwash

2 tablespoons quince
  seeds
2 pints (1.15 litres)
  boiling water
1 tablespoon sherry

Put the quince seeds into a saucepan and add the boiling water. Cover and leave to simmer over a low heat for ten minutes. When cool, add the sherry. Bottle and label.

Quince seeds have long been known for their healing properties. They are used to cure ulcerated mouths and various throat infections.

Rosemary and Mint Mouthwash

2 teaspoons
  rosemary
2 teaspoons mint
1 pint (570ml)
  boiling water
1 teaspoon tincture
  of myrrh

Place the herbs and boiling water in a saucepan, cover and leave to infuse for ten minutes. Strain. When completely cool, add the myrrh. Bottle, shake well and label.

Concentrated Mixed Spice Mouthwash

1 tablespoon ground
  nutmeg
1 tablespoon ground
  cloves
½ tablespoon
  crushed caraway
  seeds
½ tablespoon
  ground cinnamon
8 tablespoons sherry
A few drops of the
  perfumed spirit of
  your choice

Place all the spices in a screw-top container and pour in the sherry. Seal tightly and leave for four to five days to macerate. Then add perfumed spirit, such as lavender, and bottle.

This mouthwash is very strong and very concentrated and it is therefore extremely economical. Add only a few drops to half a tumbler of water.

Cornflower Mouthwash

Place the cornflower heads into a saucepan, and pour the boiling water over them. Cover, and leave them to infuse for two hours. When cool, add the myrrh. Pour into a clear glass bottle and label.

This beautiful cornflower blue liquid looks so inviting that it encourages one to use it immediately!

1 handful cornflower blooms
1 tesapoonful tincture of myrrh
3 pints (1.7 litres) boiling water

Spearmint Mouthwash

Mix all the ingredients together, bottle in an attractive airtight container and shake well.

Myrrh is little used in the average household, which is a great pity, because this stimulating antiseptic is very useful in curing gum boils and mouth ulcers.

Some years ago when I was working flat out for very long periods, I developed my first and only mouth sore. I tried almost everything, to no avail, but within a day or two of applying some tincture of myrrh, straight from the bottle, the sore had dried considerably; within a week it had healed completely. Tincture of myrrh is also extremely effective in strengthening weak, pappy gums.

11 tablespoons eau de cologne
7½ teaspoons water
6 teaspoons glycerine
2 teaspoons tincture of myrrh
2 teaspoons borax
Mint (or any other flavour) essence, quantity as desired

Witch Hazel Mouthwash

Mix the ingredients together and bottle.

When I want a simple yet refreshing mouthwash in a hurry I turn to this recipe because it's inexpensive and takes only a minute to make. The quantities given above produce over half a pint (600ml), but you can double or treble them if you wish.

Once it is bottled, I usually add either a few sprigs of mint — any type will do — or lots of lemon peel. The mint and peel may be replenished after a few days to maintain the lovely clean taste and fragrance.

15 tablespoons water
3 tablespoons witch hazel

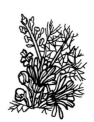

LIP GLOSSES AND SALVES

Almond Oil Lip Salve

3 teaspoons
shredded beeswax
3 teaspoonsful
almond oil

Place the beeswax in a small double boiler on a low heat and melt it slowly. Stir in the almond oil and pour the blended ingredients into a small heat-resistant mould. Once set, it should be generously applied to cracked lips.

Cocoa Butter Lip Gloss

½ teaspoon
shredded beeswax
6 teaspoons cocoa
butter

Place the beeswax in a small double boiler, melt it over a low heat and blend in the cocoa butter. Continue to stir until the mixture is liquid and pour into a small heat-resistant mould.

When the gloss has set hard, use a lip brush to apply a generous quantity evenly over the lips. It will give them a super shine!

Lanolin Lip Salve

3 teaspoons lanolin
7 teaspoons paraffin
wax
10 teaspoons white
petroleum jelly

Place all the ingredients in a small double boiler or similar container and simmer slowly until completely melted. Blend thoroughly and pour into a suitable heat-resistant mould.

This is an excellent and soothing salve for sore, dry lips.

Honey Lip Salve

6 teaspoons clear
honey
4 drops rosemary
water

Blend the ingredients together. Pot up, label and apply to the chapped lips before going to bed.

Sage Lip Cream

4 teaspoons sweet
almond oil
1 teaspoon shredded
beeswax
2 teaspoons dried
sage
4 teaspoons warm
rosewater
5 drops sage oil

Put the almond oil and the beeswax together in a double boiler and simmer slowly until they have melted and mixed. Add the dried sage, stir, cover and allow to simmer for five minutes. Remove from the heat and leave to steep for two hours. Return the mixture to a low heat, strain and whip in the rosewater. Continue blending for several minutes. Remove from the heat, add the sage oil and keep stirring until the salve thickens and cools. Pot and label.

Coconut Lip Salve

In a small double saucepan, slowly melt the beeswax and coconut oil. Remove from the heat and add the almond oil. Stir and pour into a small heat-resistant mould. Once it has set hard, it may be applied generously to chapped lips.

3 teaspoons shredded beeswax
3 tesapoons coconut oil
6 drops almond oil

Castor Oil Lip Gloss

Whip the ingredients together thoroughly. Bottle and label.

9 teaspoons lanolin
1 teaspoon castor oil

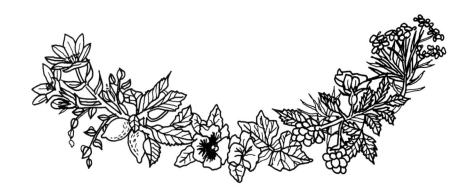

9

For the Neck

The neck is an area we frequently neglect and this is possibly why it generally shows the lines of time far earlier than the face, which is nourished twice a day.

All night and day creams should be lavishly applied to both face and throat, and some wise women cosset their necks with an additional creaming before going to bed. Extra-rich night moisturizers such as the honey anti-wrinkle night cream and the mayonnaise egg cream for wrinkles (see page 83) are excellent for this purpose. This chapter describes a few more rich skin foods which if applied to the throat regularly will help to discourage ageing lines and wrinkles.

When creaming the neck, it is important that the skin should never be pulled or stretched. Massage with gentle upward strokes starting from the base of the neck (or top of the breast if you wish) and work towards the point of the chin.

Mayonnaise and Lanolin Throat Cream

1 tablespoon lanolin
2 tablespoons mayonnaise

Warm the lanolin in a double boiler or similar container until it has melted, then whip in the mayonnaise. Remove from the heat and continue stirring until the cream is quite cold. Pot, label and refrigerate.

Apricot and Almond Throat Cream

Warm the lanolin until it melts and add the oils. Whip together, pour in the cider vinegar, remove from the heat and continue whisking until the cream has cooled. Pot and label.

2 tablespoons lanolin
2 tablespoons almond oil
1½ tablespoons apricot oil
2 teaspoons cider vinegar

Honey Throat Cream

Whip the ingredients. Pot, label and refrigerate.

Leave for twenty-four hours before applying lavishly to the throat. Gently massage into the skin. Tissue off any remaining cream after twenty minutes.

2½ tablespoons runny honey
2½ teaspoons olive oil
2 egg yolks

Cocoa Butter and Olive Oil Throat Cream

Warm the cocoa butter over a low flame. When it is melted, remove from the heat and whip in the olive oil. Stir until the mixture cools. Pot, label and refrigerate.

2 tablespoons cocoa butter
1 tablespoon olive oil

Vitamin-rich Throat Cream

Melt the lanolin in a glass bowl in a pan of hot water. Remove from the heat and add the wheatgerm, apricot kernel and carrot oils. Stir in the powdered lecithin, a little at a time, before adding the mineral water. Continue mixing until smooth and creamy. Pot up, label and refrigerate.

This rich and satiny cream with oils and natural vitamins is fine enough to be readily absorbed into the relatively thin throat skin; it is also good for thin skin around the eyes.

1 tablespoon lanolin
½ tablespoon wheatgerm oil
½ tablespoon apricot kernel oil
½ tablespoon carrot oil
1 teaspoon lecithin powder
2 teaspoons mineral water

10

For the Hair

SHAMPOOS

Willow and Birch Conditioning Shampoo

1½ handfuls fresh birch leaves
1½ handfuls fresh willow leaves
3 pints (1.7 litres) boiling water
6 tablespoons castile soap, shredded
Cider vinegar

Place the birch and willow leaves in boiling water, stir, cover and allow to infuse for two hours. Strain and add the soap. Place on a low heat and whisk constantly until the soap has melted and the mixture is smooth and creamy. Once cool, bottle and label it. Leave to stand for twenty-four hours. Remember to shake well before use.

To obtain the best results wash and rinse the hair thoroughly once and then massage more shampoo into the scalp and down the hair. Leave for ten minutes. Rinse several times with clear water, finishing with a mixture of eight parts soft water to one part cider vinegar.

Birch leaves are well known for their hair-conditioning properties, whilst willow leaves promote strong hair growth.

Together they make a worthwhile natural shampoo that is suitable for all types of hair. When used regularly, in conjunction with a conditioner, this shampoo will help prevent split ends and repair damaged hair beyond your expectations. If you need a very high-protein shampoo, beat an egg or two into the cooled mixture before bottling.

Nowadays a good soapy lather is often considered to be essential in a shampoo. Although it gives the impression of removing grime, and feels nice, it is not necessary in all shampoos and is certainly no measure of their cleansing ability. So here are two good, no-nonsense shampoos, one for blondes and one for brunettes, both of which will be appreciated by those whose eyes or skin are allergic to soap suds.

Soapless Lavender Shampoo for Fair Hair

Whisk all the ingredients together. Using your fingertips, massage the foamless mixture well into the scalp and roots and through the hair itself. Rinse and repeat, this time leaving the shampoo on the hair for ten to fifteen minutes. Rinse the hair several times, condition, rinse and set.

Juice of 2 lemons
2 teaspoons lavender water
2 eggs

Soapless Rosewater Shampoo for Dark Hair

Whip all the ingredients together. Massage the soapless mixture into the scalp and along the hair. Rinse and repeat. Leave the shampoo on the hair for ten to fifteen minutes. Finally, rinse the hair several times, then condition, rinse and set in the usual way.

2 tablespoons vinegar
2 teaspoons rosewater
2 eggs

Citrus Shampoo for Greasy Hair

Puncture and slice the peel. Place in boiling water, stir, cover and allow to infuse for two hours. Strain and add the soap to the liquid. Put on a low heat and whisk continuously until the soap is dissolved. Add the juices and whisk again. Once cool, it may be bottled and labelled.

Leave to stand for twenty-four hours, and remember to shake well before use. After shampooing, always rinse the hair several times in clear water, finishing with a mixture of eight parts soft water to one part cider vinegar.

This refreshing and fruity shampoo has a natural drying effect that makes it just the thing for extra-greasy hair. However, it is unwise to use it more than once a week unless the treatment includes an enriching conditioner.

Peel of 1 lemon, 1 orange and 1 grapefruit
3 pints (1.7 litres) boiling water
6 tablespoons castile soap, shredded
2 tablespoons lemon juice
2 tablespoons orange juice
2 tablespoons grapefruit juice
Cider vinegar

Marigold High-Lighting Shampoo

*3 pints (1.7 litres)
  boiling water
1 large handful
  marigold flowers
6 tablespoons
  shredded castile
  soap*

Steep the marigold flowers in the boiling water, stir, cover, and allow to infuse for two hours. Strain, and add the soap to the liquid. Place over a low heat, and whisk continuously until all the soap has dissolved. Remove from the heat, and, when cool, bottle and label.

Leave to stand for twenty-four hours, and make a habit of shaking it well before use. Always rinse the hair several times to ensure that it is free from all soap, before conditioning, rinsing, and setting.

Marigold shampoo is really quite special for it enhances the hair of red heads, and highlights the reddish tints in the hair of many brunettes. It leaves the hair feeling silky soft!

Lecithin Egg Conditioning Shampoo for Dry and Normal Hair

*3 tablespoons
  lecithin
6 tablespoons
  shredded castile
  soap
3 eggs
3 pints (1.7 litres)
  boiling water*

Add the lecithin to the boiling water, and keep mixing until all the lumps disappear, and the lecithin is completely dissolved. Place over a low heat, add the soap, and whisk until the soap has completely dissolved. Take off the heat, and when the solution is cool, blend in the eggs, one at a time, and keep beating until the shampoo is lumpless and creamy. Whisk, bottle, and label. Leave to stand for twenty-four hours and always shake well before use.

For the best results, wet the hair before applying the shampoo. Wash twice and rinse thoroughly before massaging more of the shampoo into the scalp and along the length of hair. Leave on for ten to fifteen minutes. Rinse, first with clear tepid water, and finally with a mixture of eight parts of soft lukewarm water to one part of cider vinegar. This is a fine tonic shampoo for damaged or extra dry, lustreless hair. Try not to use artificial heating on your hair for it has a very undesirable drying effect.

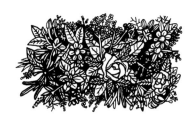

Protein-Enriched Soapwort and Orange Shampoo

Whisk the eggs and orange juice together and beat them into the infusion. Bottle, label and refrigerate.

Shampoo in the usual way, using warm water but never hot water. This is one of the best shampoos I have tried. It smells fruity and leaves the hair beautifully silky.

2 tablespoons orange juice
2 egg yolks
1 pint (570ml) extra-rich soapwort infusion (page 168)

Soapwort and Horsetail Shampoo

Place the soapwort and horsetail together in a heat-resistant bowl. Boil the soft water and pour it over the herbs. Cover and leave to infuse for twenty to twenty-five minutes. Strain, bottle and label.

Shampoo the hair in the normal way, using about half a pint (285 ml) of shampoo. Being a superb conditioner, horsetail imparts a healthy sheen as no other herb can. That is no doubt the reason it is included in the diet of Arab and other show horses.

8 tablespoons shredded soapwort root
8 tablespoons horsetail herb
4 pints (2.3 litres) soft water

Protein-Enriched Rosemary Shampoo for Dark Hair

Put the rosemary in the boiling water, stir, cover and allow to infuse for two hours. Strain and add the soap. Place on a low heat and whisk continuously until all traces of the solid soap have disappeared. Remove from the heat and blend in the borax. When completely cool, fold in the eggs and whisk until the mixture thickens. Bottle, label and leave to stand for twenty-four hours. Always shake the bottle before use.

4 tablespoons dried rosemary
3 pints (1.7 litres) boiling water
6 tablespoons castile soap, shredded
1 tablespoon borax
2 eggs

A close family friend in his late fifties regularly uses this shampoo and his thick dark brown hair is the envy of many younger men. He believes that its condition is entirely due to this shampoo. Rosemary is believed to renew and strengthen the hair, whilst keeping the scalp free from dandruff.

Camomile Shampoo for Fair Hair

3 tablespoons dried
  camomile flowers
3 pints (1.7 litres)
  boiling water
6 tablespoons castile
  soap, shredded
Juice of 1 lemon

Infuse the camomile flowers in the boiling water, stir, cover and allow to steep for two hours. Strain and add the soap to the infusion. Place over a low heat and add the lemon juice. When cool, bottle and label. Allow to stand for twenty-four hours. Remember to shake well before use. Always rinse the hair several times, using plenty of clean tepid water, before conditioning, rinsing and setting.

Protein-Enriched Sage Shampoo for Brown Hair

3 dessertspoons
  dried sage
3 pints (1.7 litres)
  boiling water
6 tablespoons castile
  soap, shredded
2 eggs
Cider vinegar

Add the sage to the boiling water, cover and allow to simmer over a low heat for twenty minutes. Strain. Add the shredded soap to the infusion. Whisk continuously until all the soap has dissolved. Remove from the heat and allow to cool. When cool, beat in the eggs, a little at a time. Whisk until well blended, bottle and leave to stand for twenty-four hours. Always shake well before use.

After shampooing, rinse thoroughly in a mixture of eight parts soft water to one part cider vinegar. Condition, rinse and set.

Herbal Anti-Dandruff Shampoo

2 handfuls fresh
  nettle tops
1½ dessertspoons
  sage
1½ dessertspoons
  thyme
3 pints (1.7 litres)
  boiling water
6 tablespoons castile
  soap, shredded

Add the nettles and other herbs to the boiling water, cover and allow to simmer for twenty minutes. Strain. Add the soap to the infusion. Whisk continuously until all the soap has dissolved and the shampoo looks rich and frothy. Remove from the heat, allow to cool, bottle and label.

After using this shampoo, always rinse the hair thoroughly, ensuring that all traces of soap have been washed away. Then condition, rinse and set. When used regularly, in conjunction with an anti-dandruff hair tonic or rub, this shampoo should keep the hair completely free of dandruff.

Anti-Dandruff Shampoo Cream

Place the glycerine and soap together in a bowl with a little of the water and allow the mixture to stand. Boil the remainder of the water, pour it over the camomile flowers and steep for thirty minutes. Strain the infusion and add the soap and glycerine. Using a wooden spoon or potato masher, warm and blend the ingredients until you have a smooth and lumpless cream. Add the oil of lemon and mix well. You should now have a stiff cream, but if it is a fraction too thick — and this could happen if you are forced to use another type of soap — add a little more boiling water. Blend and store in a screw-top jar.

1 tablespoon glycerine
12 tablespoons castile soap, shredded
16 tablespoons soft water
4 tablespoons dried camomile flowers
2 teaspoons oil of lemon

When using this cream, rub a little at a time into the scalp and hair until it is evenly covered. Massage for approximately three minutes, leave for seven minutes and then rinse. To ensure that all the soap is washed away, rinse the hair several times in water and then in a mixture of eight parts water to one part cider vinegar. Condition, rinse and set.

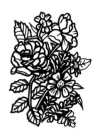

Nettle and Parsley Anti-Dandruff Shampoo

Put the parsley and the nettles in a pan of the boiling water, stir, cover and allow to steep for two hours. Strain and add the soap to the infusion. Place over a low heat and whisk until the soap has dissolved. Remove from the heat and mix in the borax. When cool, bottle and label. Leave to stand for twenty-four hours.

3 pints (1.7 litres) boiling water
1 handful fresh nettle tops
1 handful fresh parsley
6 tablespoons castile soap, shredded
1 tablespoon borax

Remember to shake well each time before use. For the best results wet the hair and work the shampoo well into the scalp and hair. Massage for three minutes, leave for a further seven minutes, then rinse, condition, rinse again and set.

Sufferers from dandruff should use this shampoo once a week without fail. After several applications even stubborn and severe cases will have improved. Nettle and parsley also help to promote strong hair growth and prevent premature hair loss.

DRY SHAMPOOS

When mixed with water, many pure, natural substances make superb shampoos. They lather well, are excellent cleansers and are themselves completely harmless but, unfortunately, after every wet shampoo the hair becomes weakened. It is not the base ingredients that cause the problem but the water itself, and it is thus advisable to use a wet shampoo no more than once a week. Too frequent washing, even of extremely greasy hair, can leave the hair fine and positively wispy!

This is where dry shampoos really are a boon! Not only do they completely eliminate these dangers but they are efficient and invaluable for all busy people. I am not suggesting that dry shampoos are substitutes for their wet counterparts, for they are not, and should never oust the regular weekly or fortnightly wash which deep-cleanses, tones and stimulates the scalp. Dry shampoos are, however, an effective means of removing grease and brushing out everyday pollution dust, and may be used frequently without any possibility of damaging or drying the hair.

Arrowroot and Orris Dry Shampoo

2 tablespoons powdered arrowroot
2 tablespoons powdered orris root

Mix the ingredients with a fork until well blended.

Massage the shampoo generously into the scalp and through the hair. Leave for thirty minutes or longer. Then brush out the powder with a clean bristle brush. Use vigorous strokes, taking care to remove all traces of shampoo from the hair and scalp. The remaining shampoo should be stored in an airtight, screw-top jar for later use.

Salt Shampoo

1 tablespoon kitchen salt

Wrap the salt in some aluminium foil and place in the oven for between five and ten minutes, until it is nicely warm. Unwrap the foil and using your fingertips massage generous quantities of the salt into the scalp and through the hair. You should then devote several minutes to brushing the now greasy salt out of the hair. Finish off with a second freshly washed brush to ensure that the last traces of dirty salt have been removed.

The salt stimulates the scalp and its quick-cleansing action leaves the hair beautifully glossy and manageable. Don't, for goodness sake, make the mistake of using table salt! When I first tried this treatment some years ago, I had run out of cooking salt and used the finer-grained table variety instead. The next hour was chaotic, as I frantically tried to brush out the fine salt particles. The awful thing is that these closely

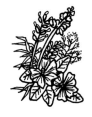

resemble dandruff and can leave your hair looking far more unkempt than when you started! The coarse-grained cooking variety will not, however, cause you any such problems.

Cornflour Meal Dry Shampoo

Massage generous quantities of the meal into the scalp and along the hair. Leave for fifteen minutes, or as long as possible if the hair is particularly greasy. Brush out thoroughly, using one brush to remove most of the meal and a second, clean one to brush away the remaining traces.

1 tablespoon cornflour meal

Hair can sparkle with vitality as can eyes and skin, but only if it is treated well. So why not finish by 'polishing' it with a silk scarf? A few minutes will give the hair such an ultra-groomed sheen that it's well worth investing in a square of silk even if you only use it as a hair polisher!

Bran and Fullers' Earth Dry Shampoo

Using a pestle and mortar, or a similar crushing tool, pulverise the bran to a coarse powder. Add the fullers' earth and blend together.

8 tablespoons bran
1 tablespoon fullers' earth powder

Massage the shampoo generously into the scalp and through the hair. Brush out with a fine bristle brush, taking care to clear all traces of powder. The remaining dry shampoo should be stored in an airtight, screw-type jar, for later use.

Salt and Orris Dry Shampoo

Mix the ingredients with a fork until they are well blended.

Massage the shampoo generously into the scalp and through the hair. Leave for thirty minutes, or longer if possible. Brush out with a clean bristle brush, using sharp strokes, and take care to remove the powder from all parts of the hair and scalp. The remaining shampoo may be stored in an airtight screw-top jar for later use.

16 tablespoons kitchen salt
1 tablespoon powdered starch
2 tablespoons powdered orris root
1 tablespoon bicarbonate of soda

This dry shampoo, using simple kitchen ingredients, has been used by women for many decades.

RINSES

Lime and Nettle Hair Rinse

1 handful lime
(linden) flowers
1 handful nettle tops
2 pints (1.15 litres)
water
2 pints (1.15 litres)
cider vinegar

Boil the lime flowers and nettles together in the water, cover and leave to simmer for ten minutes. Remove from the heat and allow to infuse for two hours. Strain and add the cider vinegar. Bottle and leave for twenty-four hours before use.

After washing your hair, add half a pint (285ml) of the liquid to the final rinse water. To gain full benefit from this invigorating rinse, soak the hair thoroughly; never dry the hair artificially but instead cover your wet hair in a warm towel until it is completely dry.

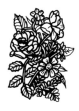

Regular use of nettle and lime stimulates the circulation and conditions the hair, leaving it beautifully soft and bouncy with lots of shine. When I met my husband he was extremely thin on top, but he experimented using a weekly conditioning shampoo, this herbal rinse and a nettle hair tonic, which he massaged nightly into his scalp. The treatment not only conditioned and strengthened what hair he had, but within three months a fine, downlike fuzz was growing on his previously bare pate! Proof indeed that these pure ingredients really do work!

Camomile and Yarrow Rinse for Fair Hair

1 handful camomile
flowers
1 handful yarrow
flowers and leaves
2 pints (1.15 litres)
boiling water
2 pints (1.15 litres)
cider vinegar

Boil the camomile and yarrow in the water, cover and simmer for seven to ten minutes. Remove from the heat and steep for a further two hours. Strain and add the cider vinegar. Bottle and leave for twenty-four hours before use.

Add half a pint (185ml) of the liquid to the final rinse water after washing your hair.

Camomile is excellent for fair hair and leaves it smelling sweet and fragrant. Yarrow helps to control excessive greasiness and prevent premature baldness. It is especially helpful in preventing and alleviating such skin problems as seborrhoea.

Comfrey and Clover Hair Rinse

Place the comfrey and clover in a quart (1.15 litre) glass jar, and add the white vinegar. Seal it with a screw-type lid, and leave it near to hand so that it can be shaken several times a day. Continue this treatment for two weeks before straining off. Approximately half a pint (185ml) of the strained liquid may be added to the final rinse water.

1 handful comfrey leaves
1 handful clover blooms
2 pints (1.15 litres) white vinegar

Comfrey acts as a natural disinfectant, and is heavenly for soothing and healing sensitive scalps.

Fruity Hair Rinse

Peel and slice the orange, apple, and melon, and puncture the orange and melon peel. Boil both the fruit and peel in the water. Cover, and allow to simmer for ten minutes. Take off the heat, and leave to stand for a further two hours. Strain, and add the cider vinegar. Bottle, and leave for twenty-four hours before use.

1 orange
1 apple
1 small slice of melon
2 pints (1.15 litres) water
2 pints (1.15 litres) cider vinegar

Wash the hair, and add half a pint (285ml) to the final rinse water.

This hair rinse is wonderfully exhilarating and refreshing to use. Like all good rinses, it restores the natural acid mantle to the hair, leaving it looking beautifully shiny, and it is superb for controlling ultra-oily locks!

Peppermint Hair Rinse

Boil the peppermint in the water, cover and simmer for ten minutes. Remove from the heat and leave to steep for an hour. Strain and add the cider vinegar. Bottle and leave for forty-eight hours before use. Having washed your hair, add half a pint (285ml) to the final rinse water.

4 heaped tablespoons dried peppermint or 8 heaped tablespoons fresh peppermint
2 pints (1.15 litres) water
2 pints (1.15 litres) cider vinegar

The natural acid which protects the hair is washed away each time the hair is shampooed; this rinse, like all other good ones, restores the essential acid balance whilst ridding the hair of all soapy particles. It leaves the hair smelling deliciously fresh and fragrant and regular use will also help prevent dandruff.

Lemon Rinse for Fair, Oily Hair

Sliced peel of 4 lemons
2 pints (1.15 litres) water
Juice of 4 lemons

Boil the lemon peel in the water, cover and simmer for ten minutes. Remove from the heat, and steep for a further two hours. Strain and add the lemon juice. Bottle. Leave for forty-eight hours before use.

After washing the hair, add half a pint (285ml) of this concoction to the final rinse water. The valuable lemon juice in this rinse restores natural acidity, while highlighting the golden tints in fair hair. The peel provides nourishing oils.

This rinse is perfect for those with oily hair, being naturally somewhat drying. Those with normal hair should therefore use only a quarter-pint in the final rinse water.

Rosemary and Sage Hair Rinse for Dark Hair

2 tablespoons dried rosemary
2 tablespoons dried sage
2 pints (1.15 litres) boiling water
¼ pint (140ml) cider vinegar

Boil the herbs in the water, cover and simmer for ten minutes. Remove from the heat, and allow to steep for two hours. Strain, add the cider vinegar and bottle. Use immediately if required.

Do not add this liquid to the final rinse water, but instead pour directly over the hair. Repeat several times, allowing the hair and scalp to absorb the rinse completely for about five minutes. Towel dry.

This is undoubtedly one of the finest of all rinses for brunettes and has long been popular. These two herbs complement each other very well. Rosemary is marvellous for preventing dandruff and adding lustre, while sage enlivens the naturally rich tints often to be found in brown hair. Together, they leave the hair smelling delightfully fresh and herby!

Onion and Lavender Hair Rinse

1 medium Spanish onion
2 pints (1.15 litres) water
2 handfuls fresh lavender heads
2 pints (1.15 litres) cider vinegar

Dice the onion and boil in the water for about fifteen minutes. Strain and add the lavender heads to the liquid. Cover and steep for two hours or until the liquid smells of lavender to your liking. Strain and add the cider vinegar. Bottle and leave for twenty-four hours before use. Add half a pint (285ml) to the final rinse water.

This may sound a somewhat bizarre hair rinse, but onions kill bacteria and help to eliminate many sorts of skin blemishes. Don't worry — your hair will not smell of onions, for the lavender will obliterate all traces of them.

Elderflower Anti-Dandruff Hair Rinse

Boil the elderflowers in the water, cover and simmer for ten minutes. Remove from the heat and infuse for an hour. Strain and add the cider vinegar. Bottle. Leave for forty-eight hours before use. After washing your hair, add half a pint (285ml) to the final rinse water.

4 handfuls fresh elderflowers
2 pints (1.15 litres) water
2 (pints (1.15 litres) cider vinegar

Elderflowers and cider vinegar both act to rid the hair of the most stubborn dandruff. Vinegar also restores the hair's protective coating and ensures that no shampoo remains to dull the hair's naturally healthy sheen. This rinse is suitable for all types of hair.

Beer Rinse for Flyaway Hair

Mix the beer and cider vinegar and bottle. This rinse may be used immediately.

2 pints (1.15 litres) draught mild or bitter beer
¼ pint (140ml) cider vinegar

Do not dilute this mixture in the final rinse water. Simply pour it directly on the head several times so that it thoroughly drenches the hair. Leave to soak and absorb the rinse for five minutes, then towel dry.

While the hair is wet, you'll smell like the inside of a brewery, but don't worry for the smell will disappear once the hair is dry. Next time you go to the pub, take a suitable screw-top bottle and bring it back filled with draught beer. I've found that this type gives far superior results, since it has more body than the weaker canned beers.

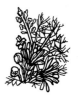

By the time you come to wash your hair the beer may have become flat and stale, but you'll find it even more effective than when it's fresh and frothy.

Yarrow and Marigold Hair Rinse

Place the yarrow and marigold blooms in a quart container, add the white vinegar and seal. Leave the container in a handy place, so that you remember to shake it several times a day. After a week, strain and remove the yarrow and marigold blooms.

1 handful yarrow
1 handful marigold heads
2 pints (1.15 litres) white vinegar

After washing the hair, add half a pint (285ml) of the liquid to the final rinse water.

I was given this country recipe by a woman who has spent much of her long life studying the uses of various herbs and flowers. As she told me, when used regularly every week, this rinse truly helps to control dandruff and combats excessively greasy hair.

Fennel Hair Rinse

2 handfuls fennel
2 pints (1.15 litres)
white vinegar

Place the fennel and white vinegar in a quart container and seal it with a screw top lid. Shake the jar several times a day, for a week. Add half a pint (285ml) of the liquid to your final rinse water after washing your hair.

This preparation is a good cleanser and instils the hair with a delightful perfume that resembles anise.

You may also like to try the following simple hair rinse infusions.

Infusion	To make
Horse tail	1 handful to 3 pints (1.7 litres) boiling water. Infuse for twenty minutes. Imparts a wonderful gloss to the hair.
Mullein (for light hair)	1 handful to 3 pints (1.7 litres) boiling water. Infuse for twenty minutes.
Nettles	1 handful to 3 pints (1.7 litres) boiling water. Infuse for twenty minutes. Helps to prevent dandruff.
Southernwood and quassia chips (for dark hair)	1 teaspoon southernwood and 2 tablespoons quassia chips to 1 pint (570ml) boiling water. Infuse for twenty five minutes.
Yarrow (for greasy hair)	1 handful to 3 pints (1.7 litres) boiling water. Infuse for twenty minutes.

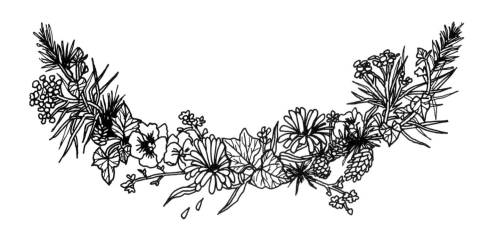

CONDITIONERS

Rum After-Shampoo Conditioner

Whisk or beat the ingredients together until well blended.

Massage the conditioner evenly into the scalp and hair for several minutes. Cover the head in a warm towel and leave for twenty-five minutes. Rinse with tepid water.

This heavenly conditioner gives the hair super body and bounce. Whether you are a blonde, brunette or redhead, it will make your hair shine like gold!

4 tablespoons rum
1 egg

Mayonnaise and Glycerine Pre-Shampoo Conditioner

Place all the ingredients in a bowl and whisk until thoroughly mixed.

Using the tips of the fingers, massage the conditioner evenly through the hair and well into the scalp. Cover the hair in a warm towel and leave for forty-five minutes or longer. Shampoo and rinse your hair in the usual way.

2 tablespoons cider vinegar
2 tablespoons glycerine
1 tablespoon olive oil
1 tablespoon coconut oil
2 eggs

Castor and Avocado Oil Pre-Shampoo Conditioner

Whisk all the ingredients together until the mixture is light and airy.

Using the fingertips, massage the conditioner evenly through the hair and well into the scalp. Wrap the hair in a towel and leave for twenty minutes. Shampoo and rinse in the usual way.

This is an enriching hair treatment for any time of the year, but you'll find it particularly beneficial when the hair lacks life and lustre. You may need it after illness, or during the hotter months when the sun, and salty sea air tend to damage and dry the healthiest of hair.

2 tablespoons avocado oil
1 tablespoon castor oil
1 teaspoon rum
2 eggs

Yogurt After-Shampoo Conditioner for Flyaway Hair

6 tablespoons
  natural yogurt
1 egg

Place the ingredients in a bowl and whisk until thoroughly blended.

Massage the conditioner evenly into the scalp and hair for four minutes. Wrap the hair in a warm towel and leave for ten to fifteen minutes. Rinse with tepid water.

This recipe was given to me years ago by a farmer's wife, who had long thick hair which always looked wonderfully tidy and well groomed. She attributed it solely to this conditioning treatment, which she employed without fail after every shampoo.

Garlic and Castor Oil Pre-Shampoo Conditioner

8 tablespoons hot
  castor oil
8 large cloves of
  garlic

Peel, slice and crush the garlic and add to the hot castor oil. Cover and steep for thirty-six hours. Strain and bottle.

Massage the conditioner evenly through the hair with the fingers, concentrating particularly on the scalp. Wrap the hair in a warm towel and leave for at least an hour, or longer if possible. Shampoo and rinse.

Being a strong antiseptic, this hair conditioner is excellent for revitalizing dry, lifeless hair. It is also a wonderful tonic for hair if you have recently been very ill. It helps prevent hair loss and seborrhoea.

Sesame and honey Pre-Shampoo Conditioner

2 dessertspoons
  sesame oil
1 teaspoonful clear
  honey
1 egg

Place all the ingredients in a bowl and whisk for several minutes, until the honey has become integrated and the conditioner nice and smooth.

Massage the conditioner evenly through the hair, concentrating on the scalp, and the dry ends of the hair. Wrap the hair in a warm towel, and leave for thirty minutes, longer if possible. Shampoo and rinse.

A terrific pick-me-up conditioner for dry and unruly hair.

Vitamin and Protein Pre-Shampoo Conditioner

Place the first five ingredients and the contents of the vitamin capsule in a bowl and whisk until thoroughly blended.

Massage the conditioner evenly through the hair, concentrating particularly on the scalp. Wrap the hair in a warm towel and leave for five to ten minutes. Shampoo and rinse.

Regular use of this recipe will make your hair much more manageable and will leave it looking lustrous and luxuriant.

1 egg
1 tablespoon castor oil
1 tablespoon almond/corn oil
1 teaspoon cider vinegar
! teaspoon glycerine
Vitamin A (10,000iu capsule)

Avocado After-Shampoo Conditioner

Mash the ingredients together with a fork, and then whisk the mixture until it is light and frothy.

Using the fingertips, massage the conditioner into the scalp and along the hair, concentrating on the dry, brittle ends of the hair. Continue this gently stimulating massage for about five minutes. Leave for a further fifteen minutes, before rinsing off with lots of lukewarm water. Towel dry, and set in the usual way.

If it were possible to buy a rich and completely pure conditioner such as this one, it would cost a small fortune! But you can treat your hair to this really luxurious conditioner for a matter of pence!

½ avocado (peeled)
½ teaspoon avocado oil
2 egg yolks

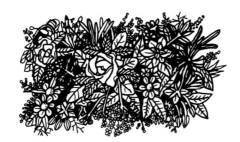

High Protein After-Shampoo Conditioner for Brittle Hair

1 dessertspoon
  wheatgerm oil
1 dessertspoon castor
  oil
2 dessertspoons olive
  oil
1 dessertspoon
  safflower oil
1 dessertspoon
  almond oil
1 dessertspoon cider
  vinegar
1 dessertspoon
  dissolved lecithin
2 eggs

Place all the ingredients in a bowl, and whisk together until well mixed.

With the fingertips, massage the conditioner evenly through the hair, and into the scalp, and continue for approximately four minutes. Wrap the hair in a warm towel, and leave for thirty minutes. Rinse with tepid water.

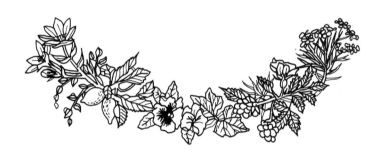

Egg and Olive Oil Pre-Shampoo Conditioner

2 tablespoons olive
  oil
1 tablespoon cider
  vinegar
1 egg yolk

Place the ingredients in a bowl, and whisk for several minutes until the conditioner is smooth.

Using the tips of the fingers, massage the conditioner evenly through the hair, concentrating particularly on the scalp and dry ends of the hair. Crown your glory with a warm towel, and leave for thirty minutes, longer if possible, then shampoo and rinse.

You can also make an easy pre-shampoo conditioner by warming either castor oil, coconut oil, linseed oil, olive oil or vegetable oil.

TONICS AND LOTIONS

A good hair tonic, used daily, keeps the hair thick, glossy and in tip-top condition. Tonics strengthen and stimulate hair growth, help keep the scalp clean and fresh and many both prevent and rid the hair of dandruff or seborrhoea. However, to be effective they must be used regularly, and it is vital to massage the chosen lotion gently into the scalp and hair rather than simply rubbing it in quickly.

Southernwood Tonic

Pour the boiling water over the southernwood leaves, cover and simmer for ten minutes. Add the wine vinegar and allow to steep for forty-eight hours. Strain, bottle and label.

This is one of my favourite hair tonics, for it has a luscious, lemony perfume and is bracing and refreshing. It serves a dual purpose: when I'm feeling exhausted, I pour about half a pint (285ml) of this infusion and a little cider vinegar into my bath water and after ten minutes' soaking I feel relaxed and rejuvenated!

2 pints (1.15 litres) boiling water
2 handfuls southernwood leaves
2 pints (1.15 litres) white wine vinegar

Anti-Dandruff Pine Hair Lotion

Make an infusion by placing the comfrey in the boiling water. Cover, and leave to simmer for two to three minutes. Remove from the heat, and allow to infuse for two hours. Add two tablespoons of this concoction to the eau de cologne and pine oil. Bottle, shake several times, and label.

2 tablespoons comfrey
½ pint (285ml) boiling water
8 tablespoons pine oil
4 tablespoons eau de cologne

Green Leaf Hair Tonic

Boil the leaves in the water for five minutes. Take off the heat, and allow to steep for two hours. Strain, add the alcohol, shake, bottle, and label.

This is the chlorophyll tonic which is just a super example of how plants, when given the opportunity, will provide us with the materials we require. Although this recipe is almost as old as the earth from which the box and southernwood spring, it is no less effective now than it was so very long ago.

8 tablespoons green box leaves
8 tablespoons green southernwood leaves
½ pint (285ml) water
4 drops alcohol

Nettle Tonic

1 pint (570ml)
  boiling water
1 handful nettle tops
1 pint (570ml) white
  wine vinegar

Pour the boiling water over the nettle tops, cover and simmer for fifteen minutes. Remove from the heat, add the white wine vinegar and steep for one hour. Filter, bottle and label.

This is a good rejuvenating tonic that I wholeheartedly recommend. If you dislike its nettle aroma, as some people do, add a little eau de cologne when you use it.

Antiseptic Birch Tonic

1 large clove of
  garlic
1 pint (570ml) eau
  de cologne
1 small handful
  birch leaves
¾ pint (425ml)
  boiling water

Peel and chop the garlic and steep in the eau de cologne for four days. On the third day, make an infusion of the birch leaves with the boiling water, cover and simmer for ten minutes. Remove from the heat and allow to steep for a further twenty-four hours. On the fourth day, strain the birch liquid and the garlic eau de cologne and pour the two into a screw-top bottle. Shake several times and label.

Garlic is renowned as a first-class antiseptic and, like the birch leaves is believed to stimulate vigorous hair growth.

Hair Tonic with Chillies

4 small sliced
  chillies
1 pint (570ml) eau
  de cologne

Steep the chopped chillies in the eau de cologne for seven days. Strain, bottle and label.

Chillies are used in many mass-produced hair lotions because they activate the hair roots and thus help prevent seborrhoea and excessive hair loss.

Castor Oil Hair Lotion with Chillies

3 small chillies,
  diced
12 tablespoons
  alcohol
9 teaspoons castor
  oil
6 teaspoons rum

Steep the chillies in the alcohol for four days. Add the other ingredients and leave to stand for a further twenty-four hours. Strain, bottle and label.

This enriching and stimulating lotion may be applied four or five times a week when the hair is very dry, brittle and in generally poor condition. Normal hair will also benefit from applications of this conditioning lotion, once or twice a week being more than sufficient.

Willow and Mace Hair Tonic

Pour the rectified spirit into a medium-sized jar and add as many crushed willow leaves as the jar will take. Seal tightly and shake daily for ten days. After this time has elapsed, strain off the spirit and pour it with all the other ingredients into a double boiler. Heat very gently, stirring constantly, until the mixture is thoroughly blended. Bottle and label.

Massage this wonderful tonic into the scalp daily.

*2 tablespoons
rectified spirit
Willow leaves,
crushed
1 tablespoon mace
oil
4 drops rosemary oil
4 drops carbonate of
ammonia solution*

Romany Hair Lotion

Steep the onion in the rum for thirty-six hours. Strain, bottle and label.

I have only met a few true Romanies, but they all possessed beautiful blue-black hair, which shone as brightly as their highly polished and much-prized copper ornaments. The recipe for this conditioning lotion was given to me by one such Romany years ago and could be the secret behind those long braids of thick, glossy hair!

*8 tablespoons rum
1 diced medium-
sized juicy onion*

Yarrow Hair Tonic

Pour the boiling water over the yarrow, cover and simmer for ten to fifteen minutes. Add the wine vinegar and infused for twenty-four hours. Strain, bottle and label.

Yarrow is rich in vitamins. It imparts a spicy aroma to the lotion, which helps chase away milder forms of dandruff and prevent premature baldness. It conditions and generally improves the overall appearance of all types of hair.

*2 pints (1.15 litres)
boiling water
2 handfuls yarrow
leaves and flowers
2 pints (1.15 litres)
white wine
vinegar*

Quince Hair Tonic

Place the peel in the water, cover and heat slowly for fifteen minutes. Do not bring to the boil. Remove from the heat and allow the contents to infuse for about eight hours. Strain, bottle and label.

*2 handfuls quince
peel, diced
1 pint (570ml) water*

Lime and Horsetail Hair Tonic

Place the herbs in the water, cover and heat slowly for fifteen minutes. Do not bring to the boil. Remove from the heat and allow to stew overnight. Strain, bottle and label.

*1 handful horsetail
stems
1 handful lime
(linden) flowers
1 pint (570ml) water*

SETTING LOTIONS AND GELS

Quince Seed Setting Lotion and Gel

2 teaspoons quince
seeds
8 tablespoons boiling
water

Put the seeds into the water, cover and allow to infuse for three hours. Strain, bottle and label.

A thicker setting gel may be produced by simmering the seeds in the water. As they break up, a further teaspoon of seeds may be added. Repeat several times until the liquid becomes a thick jelly. Strain and leave to cool. Pot and label.

These lotions are particularly useful, for as well as keeping the hair neat and well groomed the quince extract feeds and nurtures the hair. In this respect the lotion is unlike some mass-produced setting lotions, which cause extreme dryness and in some cases actual damage. Quince seeds contain a substance which is renowned in some countries for promoting healthy and luxuriant hair growth.

Quickie Setting Lotion with Sugar

1 tablespoon sugar
8 tablespoons warm
water

Dissolve the sugar in the water and still well. Pour the solution into a bottle or atomizer.

There is a choice of ways in which to use this setting lotion. It may be combed through the hair before you set it or sprayed on once the hair has been dressed. It is fairly tacky and sticky and the hair will need to be shampooed after twenty-four hours, but it is a good standby in an emergency.

I would recommend that this lotion be used only during the winter months, for insects attracted to the sugar could prove a nuisance in the summer.

Egg Setting Lotion

1 tablespoon raw
egg white
4 tablespoons warm
water

Whisk the ingredients for several minutes until the lotion is well balanced. Bottle, label and refrigerate.

Comb the lotion through the hair and set in the usual way.

Glycerine and Alcohol Setting Lotion

Soak the tragacanth in the glycerine and water for twenty-four hours. Transfer the mixture to a pan and warm over a low flame, stirring all the time. When the ingredients are thoroughly mixed, remove from the heat. When cool, add the alcohol. Whisk for a minute or more and then bottle and label.

¼ tablespoon gum tragacanth
1½ tablespoons of glycerine
1¼ (700ml) water
5 tablespoons alcohol

Simple Brilliantine

Pour all the ingredients into a bottle. Cork and shake vigorously until the oils and alcohol have merged. Label.

This brilliantine appears somewhat pricey at first, but just calculate how much this amount of the shop-bought type would cost and you'll discover that you are definitely on to a winner.

1 pint (570ml) alcohol
¼ pint (140ml) castor oil
A few drops of your favourite aromatic oil

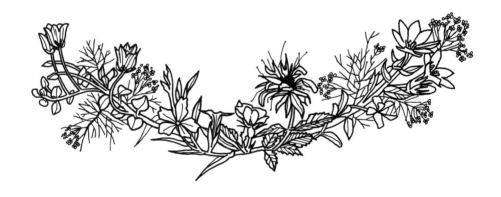

COLOURANTS AND DYES

Colouring or dyeing the hair is a very personal affair. Nowadays an increasing number of women want to break with the modern practice of using chemicals to colour the hair, and revert to older and safer techniques that use vegetable dyes.

It can be thrilling to experiment with the colourants in this section, but there is one point that I must emphasize. To achieve a specific shade of gold, red, brown or whatever will now involve more than simply visiting the chemist's, and choosing a shade with the help of a colour chart. With vegetable dyes, no such guidelines are available. At first, all you can do is experiment by making up a solution that is weaker than necessary and testing it on a strand of hair hidden behind your ears. If, when dry, the treated section does not have the required tint, you can reduce or increase the strength of the solution as appropriate. It is very much a matter of trial and error, but this can prove a lot of fun! Always remember to do that simple test beforehand and you can't go wrong!

When using any dye, make sure that your hands are protected with rubber gloves. It's the colour of your hair you want to change — not your hands!

Sage Tea Rub to Mask Grey Hair

2 teaspoons dried
  sage
2 teaspoons India
  tea
1 pint (570ml) soft
  water
2 teaspoons rum

Place the sage and tea together in a pan and add the water. Bring to the boil, cover, and simmer over a low flame for about two hours. Remove from the heat and let the mixture cool. Strain it and stir in the rum. Bottle and label.

Rub this solution into the scalp five times a week to help mask premature greying of the hair.

Elderberry Hair Rinse to Enrich Grey Hair

16 tablespoons
  elderberries
1 pint (570ml) water

Make an infusion by boiling and simmering the elderberries and water together for forty-five minutes. Strain and bottle.

To enrich grey hair with a beautiful, soft bluish tone, rinse the hair in this solution after shampooing. If necessary repeat several times until the right shade is achieved.

A stronger solution using more elderberries makes a perfect hair rinse for those who wish to give their black hair a darker, bluish and more brilliant shine.

Tobacco Solution to Darken Grey Hair

Steep the tobacco in the boiling water for thirty minutes. Strain and bottle. Pour the rinse over the hair. Repeat the treatment daily until the hair is the required colour.

4 teaspoons dark tobacco
10 tablespoons boiling water

Camomile Lightening Paste

Make an infusion by immersing the camomile heads in boiling water and simmering for twenty-five minutes. When cool, strain off a half-pint (285ml) of liquid and stir in the kaolin powder and egg yolk. Apply to the hair and leave on for between twenty and fifty minutes. Rinse with warm water. Several applications may be needed to achieve the desired fair tone.

5 tablespoons camomile heads
¾ pint (425ml) soft water
8 tablespoons kaolin powder
1 egg yolk

Rhubarb and Camomile Lightening Rinse for Blonde Hair

Make an infusion by boiling and simmering the rhubarb and camomile together for approximately twenty-five minutes. When cool, stir in the borax. Strain, and bottle.

Add ½ pint (285ml) to the final rinse water after shampooing, and immerse your hair in it. Repeat the treatment on successive days until you achieve the desired shade.

4 tablespoons chopped rhubarb
4 tablespoons camomile
1½ tablespoons borax
1 pint (570ml) soft water

Rhubarb Lightening Paste

Make an infusion by boiling and then simmering the stem, root and water together for twenty-five minutes. When cool, strain off half a pint (285ml) of the infusion, and stir in the kaolin powder, and then the egg yolk, vinegar and glycerine. Apply to the hair and leave for between twenty and fifty minutes, depending on the depth of colour you require. Rinse off with warm water. It will lighten fair and brown hair to varying shades of gold, but several applications may be necessary before you achieve the desired tint.

2 tablespoons crushed rhubarb root and stem
¾ pint (425ml) soft water
8 tablespoons kaolin powder
1 egg yolk
½ teaspoon cider vinegar
1 teaspoon glycerine

Mullein Golden Rinse

5 tablespoons
 mullein leaves
¾ pint (425ml) soft
 water

Make an infusion by boiling the leaves in water and then simmering for twenty-five minutes. When cool, strain and bottle.

After shampooing, rinse your hair in the infusion. Repeat the treatment more than once, until the hair takes on the desired shade of gold.

Walnut Paste (for Browner Hair)

6 tablespoons green
 walnut skins
6 tablespoons
 orangeflower
 water
5 teaspoons
 powdered alum
1 egg yolk

Chop the walnut skins very finely, add the orangeflower water, alum and egg yolk, and mix to a smooth paste. Apply the paste evenly to the hair. Leave for between thirty minutes and one hour depending on your natural hair colour and the shade of brown you require. Shampoo in the usual way. Sometimes more than one application is needed for the required results.

Henna Rinse (for Browner Hair)

2 tablespoons henna
 powder
1 pint (570ml) water

Make an infusion by boiling the henna in water and simmering for about ten minutes. Strain and bottle.

This is an excellent conditioning rinse as well as a soft colourant. Even those who have never experimented with dyes before will find that this rinse is reliable — and so you can't go terribly wrong. Rinse the hair in this solution after shampooing. Several rinse may be necessary before the right tone is achieved.

Indigo and Henna Paste (for Blacker Hair)

8 tablespoons henna
22 tablespoons
 pounded indigo
 leaves
Boiling water
1 egg yolk
Corn oil

Mix the henna and indigo with sufficient boiling water to make a smooth paste. When cool, stir in the egg yolk. Massage plenty of corn oil into the scalp to prevent the hair becoming dry and then apply the paste evenly to the hair. Leave for between one and two hours depending on your hair colour and the shade of black required.

If you find that this recipe does not give you blue-black hair reduce the quantity of henna and leave the paste on longer until you achieve the correct shade. Shampoo in the usual way.

Walnut and Rosemary Rub (for Black Hair)

Macerate the skins in the alcohol, seal and leave for ten to twelve days. Strain. Beat in the rosemary oil. Bottle and label.

Having dried your freshly shampooed hair, massage the alcohol rub evenly through the hair and into the scalp. If applied regularly, it will gradually darken the hair and prevent the roots from showing signs of premature greying.

8 tablespoons green walnut skins
8 tablespoons alcohol
A few drops rosemary oil

Hibiscus Rinse to Redden Hair

Make an infusion by boiling the hibiscus blooms in the water and simmering for ten minutes. Remove from the heat and leave for one hour. Strain and bottle.

After shampooing, rinse the hair in this infusion to highlight the reddish tones often present in brown hair.

1 handful hibiscus heads
1 pint (570ml) water

Henna and Lemon Paste to Redden Hair

Mix the henna, ground coffee and lemon juice, and add enough boiling water to make a paste. Leave to stand for thirty minutes.

Meanwhile, massage some corn oil into the scalp to prevent drying. After the necessary time has elapsed, beat the egg into the henna mixture and apply the paste evenly to the hair. Depending on the natural tone of your hair and the rich auburn tint that you want, leave the paste on for one to one and a half hours. Shampoo in the usual way.

10 tablespoons Iranian henna
1 tablespoon ground coffee
Juice of 2 lemons
Boiling water
Corn oil
1 egg yolk

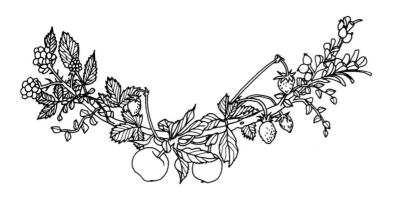

11

For the Hands and Nails

MOISTURIZING CREAMS, LOTIONS AND GELS

Coconut Hand Cream

3 tablespoons
  shredded beeswax
4 tablespoons sweet
  almond oil
4 tablespoons
  coconut oil
6 tablespoons
  glycerine

Place the wax, almond and coconut oils together in a double saucepan or similar utensil over a low heat. Melt and blend together. Add the glycerine slowly, drop by drop, and keep stirring until the ingredients become one mass of smooth, silky cream. Pot and label.

Almond Hand Jelly

8 tablespoons white
  petroleum jelly
8 tablespoons
  lanolin
2 tablespoons
  almond oil
2 tablespoons
  rosewater

Warm the petroleum jelly in a double saucepan until it is runny, remove from the heat and add the lanolin. Beat well until the mixture becomes somewhat creamy in texture. Pour in the almond oil, a few drops at a time, beating continuously. Mix in the rosewater in the same way. Whip for several minutes and leave to stand for eight hours. Whisk again, pot and label.

Cornflour Hand Cream

Place the glycerine in a double boiler over a low heat and beat in the cornflour a little at a time. Stir until the mixture changes to a smooth paste. Add the rosewater, a few drops at a time, and stir until the consistency becomes firm and creamy. Pot and label.

This extremely pure cream may be applied to the most sensitive skin without causing any irritation.

2 tablespoons glycerine
2 tablespoons cornflour
½ pint (285ml) rosewater

Tomato Hand Lotion

Beat all the ingredients together. Bottle, shake well, label and refrigerate. Apply lavishly at any time. Use up within two to three days.

Juice of 1 over-ripe tomato
1 teaspoon glycerine
1 teaspoon lemon juice

Elderflower and Camomile Hand Gel

For this recipe I suggest that you use a fairly large quantity of petroleum jelly, for only then may a sufficient quantity of elderflowers and camomile be absorbed.

Warm the petroleum jelly in a double boiler or similar receptacle, and then stir in equal quantities of elderflower and camomile until the runny jelly is packed to full capacity. Continue stirring all the time. Cover and simmer over a low heat for forty-five minutes. Strain, pot and label.

Petroleum jelly
Elderflowers, coarsely chopped
Camomile flowers, coarsely chopped

Honey Hand Lotion

Warm the honey gently over a low heat until it runs easily. Remove from the heat and blend in the other ingredients. Whisk well, bottle and label.

1½ teaspoons clear honey
10 tablespoons rosewater
4 tablespoons glycerine
½ teaspoon white vinegar

Bran Hand Lotion for Rough Hands

1 pint (570ml)
boiling water
1 handful bran
flakes
4 tablespoons cider
vinegar

Pour the boiling water over the bran, cover and leave to infuse for eight to twelve hours. Strain and add the cider vinegar. Stir well, bottle and label.

This is a non-greasy hand lotion that works wonders with rough and chapped hands. It should be applied whenever possible throughout the day. Rub it into the hands until they feel quite dry.

Non-greasy Hand Lotion

1 teaspoon witch
hazel
½ tablespoon
glycerine
3 tablespoons eau de
cologne

Mix the witch hazel and glycerine, and stir. Add the eau de cologne. Shake well, bottle and label.

This gentle, no-nonsense hand lotion is wonderfully practical for it can be applied as often as you wish and it never leaves the hands feeling sticky or greasy. Rub a few drops at a time into the hands until they feel absolutely dry.

Groundsel Hand Lotion

8 tablespoons
chopped groundsel
5 tablespoons
glycerine
2½ pints (1.4 litres)
soft water
10 tablespoons
alcohol

Leave the goundsel and glycerine in the water for thirty-six hours. Next, place them in a saucepan, cover and simmer over a low heat for fifteen minutes. Remove from the heat and leave to infuse for forty-eight hours. Strain and stir in the alcohol. Blend thoroughly, bottle and label.

This is one of the most soothing and healing of all hand lotions and should be applied frequently and generously to very sore and badly chapped hands. You'll find that its healing qualities are quite surprising.

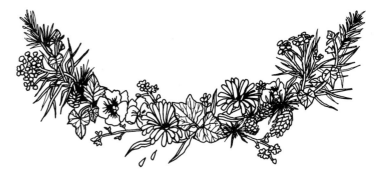

Extra-enriching Night Oil for Dehydrated Hands

Warm the honey in a double boiler or similar receptacle. When runny, add the oils and glycerine. Whip for several minutes until completely blended. Pot and label.

Apply this rich oil generously to the hands last thing at night. Rub it in for several minutes, before donning a pair of old cotton gloves. You'll notice the difference after just one application.

1 teaspoon clear honey
2 tablespoons olive oil
1 tablespoon sesame oil
1 tablespoon almond oil
½ tablespoon glycerine

Brandy Cucumber Hand Lotion

To the finely mashed cucumber, add the glycerine, brandy and rosewater. Whisk the ingredients thoroughly for several minutes until they are well blended. Pot and label.

This is a good moisturizer and is delightfully cooling and invigorating to use.

Years ago, having made a small quantity, I realized just how good this hand lotion was and started to make regular quantities in the late afternoons when I was alone. Over a period of weeks, my husband noticed that small but regular quantities of his after-dinner brandy were disappearing. It took a lot of effort to convince him that I was pouring it on my hands and not down my throat!

2 tablespoons cucumber, peeled and mashed
2 tablespoons glycerine
2 tablespoons brandy
2 tablespoons rosewater

Great-Grandmother's Hand Lotion

Using a pestle or similar crushing tool, pound the powdered tragacanth until all the lumps have disappeared. Add the glycerine and stir the mixture until it becomes a stiff, smooth paste. Next, pour in the rosewater and eau de cologne a few drops at a time until half of each remains. All these ingredients must be well blended together. Then put the camphor in the remaining eau de cologne and pour the liquid a little at a time into the creamy mixture.

Then add the remaining rosewater and the hydrogen peroxide to make a fine emulsion. If you find the lotion a little too thick for your needs, add a few extra drops of rosewater. Bottle and label.

½ teaspoon powdered gum tragacanth
1 tablespoon glycerine
8 tablespoons rosewater
2 tablespoons eau de cologne
5 drops spirit of camphor
1 tablespoon hydrogen peroxide

Victorian Hand Lotion for Chapped Hands

¼ teaspoon
  powdered gum
  tragacanth
1 tablespoon
  glycerine
1 tablespoon clear
  honey
24 teaspoons
  rosewater
¼ teaspoon borax
A little boiling water
½ teaspoon liquid
  ammonia
A few drops of oil of
  lemon

Crush the powdered gum tragacanth with the glycerine, add the honey and a few drops of rosewater and stir for several minutes. Dissolve the borax in a small quantity of boiling water and add the ammonia. Pour this liquid, a few drops at a time, into the gum and glycerine mixture. Add the remaining rosewater. When the mixture is completely smooth, add the oil of lemon. You now have a soothing and satinlike lotion, but if you prefer it a little thinner, stir in a small quantity of boiled and cooled water. Bottle and label.

Potato and Glycerine Hand Lotion

1 tablespoon fresh
  lemon juice
3 teaspoons
  glycerine
1 teaspoon strained
  potato water
10 drops tincture of
  benzoin

Add the lemon juice to the glycerine and then add the potato water. Blend the tincture of benzoin drop by drop — keep whisking until well mixed otherwise the concoction may curdle. Bottle and shake thoroughly a few times before labelling.

This very simple and inexpensive lotion is wonderful for whitening and softening the hands and should be applied generously several times a day.

Fruity Hand Lotion

3 tablespoons
  rosewater
3 tablespoons
  glycerine
3 tablespoons
  alcohol
1 tablespoon lemon
  juice
1 tablespoon orange
  juice
1 tablespoon cider
  vinegar

Mix all the ingredients together. Bottle, shake well and label.

Each time we wash our hands we remove the vital acids which act as a protective shield for the skin. The fruit contained in this lotion is beneficial because it restores this natural acidity. If applied regularly after washing, this lotion will leave the hands looking white and well cared for.

Almond Hand Balm

With a pestle or similar crushing tool, pound the almonds with a little rosewater, until the rosewater looks nice and milky. Strain the liquid through gauze or muslin. Next, pound the castile soap with the glycerine and the remainder of the rosewater. Pour the two liquids into a large bottle. Shake well and add the almond essence drop by drop.

The balm is very soothing and helps to moisturize and whiten the most houseworn of hands.

8 tablespoons sweet almonds, grated
12 tablespoons rosewater
½ teaspoon castile soap, finely grated
½ teaspoon glycerine
½ teaspoon almond essence

Egg Barrier Cream

Mix the ingredients together to form a paste.

Rub into the hands and over and under the nails, and leave to dry. Once your heavy work is completed, wash off the remainder of the cream. Such a cream is, I think, far superior to those sold in the shops, because it not only protects but also nourishes the hands with nature's own moisturizers.

1 teaspoon fullers' earth
1 teaspoon sunflower oil
1 egg yolk

Jasmine Hand Gel

Slowly warm the glycerine in a double boiler or something similar, and add the arrowroot. Pour in the warmed jasmine water, and keep stirring until the mixture clears. Allow the gel to cool before storing it in a screw-top jar.

This fragrant non-spill hand gel makes a good practical travelling companion and it is delightful and easy to apply.

1 tablespoon glycerine
1 tablespoon powdered arrowroot
8 tablespoons jasmine water

Maize Hand Whitening Cream

Pound the meal and flour together, adding sufficient rosewater to make the mix into a good stiff paste. Add the benzoin and the peroxide of hydrogen, stir well, and pot up in a screw-top jar, and label.

A natural cream which, as its name suggests, has a desirable bleaching effect on the hands, whilst acting as a good and very practical barrier cream. Because it is unscented, and mainly comprised of ordinary edible foods, I usually keep a jar in the kitchen so that it's close at hand whenever I need it!

16 tablespoons almond meal
8 tablespoons maize flour
Rosewater
6 drops tincture of benzoin
10 drops peroxide of hydrogen

HAND CLEANSERS

Sugar Hand Cleanser

Castor sugar
Freshly squeezed
lemon juice

Pour a little mound of castor sugar into the palm of one hand. With the other, add the lemon juice until the sugar is thoroughly moistened. Rub this slightly abrasive mixture all over the hands and under the nails for several minutes. Rinse off with tepid water.

This treatment removes the most stubborn stains, leaving the hands white and silky soft. Whether I have any ingrained stains or not, I use this deep cleansing scrub about twice each month as an integral part of my hand care.

Oatmeal Hand Cleanser

Oatmeal
Milk

Pour a little of the meal into the palm of one hand. Add sufficient milk just to moisten it. Rub the oatmeal over the hand for some minutes and rinse with warm water. This leaves hands beautifully clean and soft.

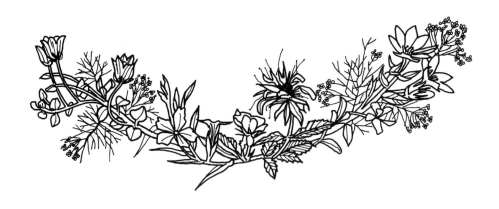

CUTICLE CREAMS AND NAIL LOTIONS

Olive Oil Nail Food

Whisk all the ingredients together, bottle and label.

Apply this food to the nails as frequently as possible, using if you wish, the same method as prescribed in the 'Protein Enriched Nail Oil' recipe. Alternatively, a very small wad of cotton wool may be soaked in the oil, and then rubbed on and around the nails.

3 teaspoons olive oil
3 teaspoons cider vinegar
1 egg yolk

Lanolin Cuticle Cream

Melt all the ingredients in a double boiler over a low flame, stirring all the time. Remove from the heat and continue stirring until the cream has thickened and cooled. Pot and label.

8 tablespoons white petroleum jelly
1 teaspoon lanolin
¼ teaspoon beeswax

Lecithin Cuticle Cream

Mix ingredients to form a smooth paste. Pot and label.

2 tablespoons pure lanolin
2 teaspoons lecithin powder

Lemon and Iodine Nail Lotion

Mix the ingredients together, bottle and label.

A small brush — an old lip brush will do nicely — dipped into this lotion and then applied to the nails several times a day (particularly first thing in the morning and late at night) will help to strength them considerably. Within a few weeks you'll begin to notice the difference.

1 teaspoon lemon juice
1 teaspoon white iodine

Protein-enriched Nail Oil

1 egg yolk
4 teaspoons sea salt
4 teaspoons castor oil
1 teaspoon runny honey
1 teaspoon wheatgerm oil

Whisk all the ingredients together, bottle and label.

I usually treat my nails to this protein oil two or three times a week. The most effective time to apply it is last thing at night.

Keep the oil in a clean, old nail varnish bottle. Then you can paint your nails in the way you apply nail varnish. Wait for the first application to dry and repeat the process several times.

Other Treatments for Strengthening the Nails

Soak them in an infusion of horsetail (1 handful to three pints/1.7 litres water), dill (1 handful to three pints/1.7 litres water) or cider vinegar (undiluted). It also helps to soak the nails in warmed olive oil, almond oil, castor oil or lanolin.

Internal treatments will also strengthen the nails. Try drinking fresh cucumber juice or eating oatmeal daily.

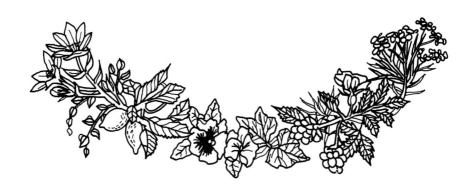

12

For the Body

BATH OILS, SOAKS AND VINEGARS

Millionairess' Beauty Bath Oil

Whip the eggs, oils and honey together. Continue whisking — all the time — while adding the alcohol, milk and soap flakes. Bottle, label and refrigerate.

Add a little at a time to your warm running bath water. Avoid using very hot water.

To my mind, even though it is without perfume this ultra-rich bath oil is far superior to anything I have found in the shops. Although more expensive to produce than other bath oils in this book, it is well worth trying — even if you have to save up to do it!

The exotic oils and high-protein eggs moisturize and feed the skin, the honey softens and soothes, the alcohol braces and stimulates, and milk is one of the oldest skin beautifiers. Even if it cost a hundred pounds to produce — which it doesn't — I think every penny would be well spent! Believe me, it really makes you feel like a million dollars!

2 eggs
16 tablespoons olive oil
8 tablespoons corn oil
8 tablespoons almond oil
3 teaspoons honey
8 tablespoons alcohol
16 tablespoons milk
2 teaspoons mild soap flakes

157

Mixed Grain Bath Powder

3 tablespoons
 kitchen salt
1 tablespoon crushed
 barley
1 tablespoon bran
2 tablesoons oatmeal
 flour
1 tablespoon ground
 almonds
1 tablespoon wheat
 flour

Blend all of the ingredients together, pot and label.

When about to bath, pour a tablespoon or so into the hand, and clench it loosely. Holding the closed fist under the tap palm upwards, allow the running water to slowly disperse the powder into the bath. Any sediment may be swished around. This mixed grain powder is a real tonic for the skin, but the best results can be obtained only if you lie back, relax and soak for about fifteen minutes.

Jasmine Bath Oil

¾ pint (425ml) of
 non-edible castor
 oil (ask the
 chemist for
 'treated' castor oil)
½ pint (285ml)
 alcohol
3–4 tablespoons
 jasmine oil

Whisk the ingredients together, bottle and label. Only a small quantity — no more than a tablespoon — is needed for each bath.

Pine Bath Soak

4 handfuls of
 crushed pine
 leaves and cones
3 pints (1.7 litres)
 boiling water

Place the bruised leaves and cones into a saucepan and pour the boiling water over them. Cover and let them simmer over a low heat for fifteen minutes. Remove from the heat and infuse for twenty-four hours. Strain, bottle, label and refrigerate.

Pour a pint (570ml) of this pine-scented essence into the bath water. Its refreshing and stimulating properties make it marvellous as a pre-party pick-me-up.

Wild Herb Bath Soak

Place the herbs into a saucepan or heat-resistant bowl and pour the boiling water over them. Cover and steep for twenty-four hours. Strain, bottle, label and refrigerate.

Add a pint (570ml) of this relaxing concoction to the bath water. The infused cowslip blooms will encourage you to sleep.

2 handfuls nettles, chopped
2 handfuls dandelions, chopped
2 handfuls cowslip heads
3 pints (1.7 litres) boiling water

Peppermint Bath Vinegar

Pour the cider vinegar and water into a saucepan and heat until the contents are almost, but not quite, boiling. Add the herbs, cover and simmer for ten minutes. Remove from the heat and leave to infuse for eight hours. Strain, bottle and label. Add half a pint (285ml) to the bath water.

1 pint (570ml) cider vinegar
1 pint (570ml) water
4 tablespoons dried peppermint
2 tablespoons dried basil

Herbal Bath Water

Put the cider vinegar and water into a saucepan. Place over a low heat and allow it to become hot without reaching boiling point. Stir in the chosen herb or herbs, cover and simmer for ten minutes. Remove from the heat and leave for eight hours. Strain, bottle and label.

Add half a pint (285ml) to the bath water.

1 pint (570ml) cider vinegar
1 pint (570ml) water
6 tablespoons chopped herbs (eucalyptus, mint, lemon balm, dandelion or elderflowers used singly or in any combination)

Alcoholic Bath Oil

Mix the brandy and oils together. Bottle, shake well and label.

This oil may seem expensive, but only a teaspoon is needed for each bath — which makes it as economical as any cheaper shop-bought product. Just think, the above quantity will provide you with enough oil for about twenty-six baths!

8 tablespoons brandy
20 drops oil of marjoram
1 teaspoon oil of thyme
20 drops of lavender

Reducing Bath Mix

8 tablespoons
  carbonate of soda
8 tablespoons borax
2 tablespoons
  glycerine
8 tablespoons
  kitchen salt
8 tablespoons
  powdered alum
3 pints (1.7 litres)
  boiling water

Place all the ingredients in a pan, and pour the boiling water over them. Keep stirring until they dissolve and then add the liquid to your warm bath water.

Wallow in the bath for twenty minutes. Stand up, wrap yourself in a thick bath towel and rub briskly all over for several minutes until your skin is completely dry and nicely toned. Get into the bath again, lie back and soak. Whilst your body is submerged, grip some flesh between your thumb and middle finger and lift it in a plucking type motion. Lift, release, lift, release, until you have treated all the fatty parts of the body. Do not, however, massage immediately on or around the breasts. Using brisk circular movements, soap and rub your body with a stiff loofah. Towel off.

This reducing bath treatment will probably make you feel somewhat tired and drained, and should, therefore, be taken only prior to retiring to bed. Many pounds may be shed. You can safely take these baths as frequently as every other day, depending on how much weight you wish to lose.

Sage Rejuvenating Bath Mix

2 pints (1.15 litres)
  boiling water
2 tablespoons dried
  sage
2 tablespoons
  kitchen salt
2 tablespoons
  bicarbonate of
  soda
2 tablespoons castile
  soap, finely grated
2 tablespoons starch

Boil the water in the saucepan, add the sage, cover and allow to simmer for fifteen minutes. Remove from the heat, and leave to infuse for an hour. Strain the liquid into another container and keep it in the bathroom for use later. Next mix the salt, soda, soap and starch.

Pour the mixture into your warm bath water. Swish the water around, get in, and soak in the water for ten to fifteen minutes. Only after this time has elapsed should the sage infusion be added. Lie back again and relax for a further fifteen minutes.

It is important that this bath mix is used in two stages. The first helps rid the body of normally acquired poisons and the second revitalizes and tones the already cleansed pores.

Honeyed Milk Beauty Bath Soak

Pour half the boiling water into a pan to which the honey has been added, and stir until the latter is completely dissolved. Add the milk and whisk. Place the salt and soda into a second container and add the remaining water. Stir. Once the salt and soda are dissolved, mix the two liquids together in a large container and shake.

Standing in a bath of warm water, rub this liquid over your feet, legs, body and arms, massaging it in for several minutes. Add a cupful to the bath water and relax for about fifteen minutes. This makes a superb bath soak because it tones and rids the skin of dead cells and softens, nourishes and soothes the body, thereby inducing restful sleep.

1½ pints (850ml) boiling water
1lb (455g) honey
1½ pints (850ml) milk
8 tablespoons kitchen salt
2 tablespoons carbonate of soda

Southernwood Bath Soak

Place the leaves in a heat-resistant pan and pour the boiling water over them. Cover and allow to steep for about one hour. Strain, bottle and label.

Pour one pint (570ml) of the infusion into the bath water and relax in the fragrant lemon-smelling water for fifteen to twenty minutes. The soak has a calming effect and I use it as a pick-me-up prior to going out for the evening.

3 handfuls chopped southernwood leaves
3 pints (1.7 litres) boiling water

Valerian and Camomile Sleep-Inducing Bath Vinegar

Place the flowers and root into a large jar and pour the boiling vinegar over them. Secure the lid and place the jar in a prominent corner to remind you to shake it several times a day. Allow to infuse for fourteen days. Strain and bottle. Use about one cupful per bath.

The ingredients contained in this recipe induce a calm, relaxed state which ensures sound sleep.

12 tablespoons camomile flowers
4 tablespoons dried valerian root
½ pint (285ml) boiling white wine vinegar

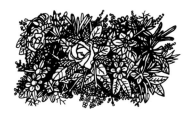

Bay Bath Vinegar

8 tablespoons
  crushed bay leaves
1 pint (570ml)
  boiling water
1 pint (570ml) cider
  vinegar

Place the bay leaves in a heat-resistant container, and over them pour the boiling water. Cover and infuse for thirty minutes. Add the cider vinegar, leave for one hour and then strain, bottle and label.

Pour about a pint (570ml) of the infusion into the bath water and immerse yourself in the herb-smelling vinegar for fifteen to twenty minutes. It seems to ease all the aches and pains of a hectic and tiring day.

Cornflower Bath Vinegar

1 pint (570ml)
  cornflower heads
1 pint (570ml)
  boiling white
  vinegar

Cram the flowers into a large screw-capped jar, and on to them pour the boiling vinegar. Secure the lid firmly, and place it in an obvious position — perhaps in the kitchen, so that it will remind you to shake it whenever you pass. Leave it to steep for fourteen days, strain, and pour into an attractive bottle which will look nice in the bathroom. Use a cupful per bath.

When I'm having a quiet soak in the warm cornflower blue water, surrounded by my evergreen pot plants, it's just like bathing in a gladed blue lagoon, and that's a tonic in itself!

Almond Bath Milk

16 tablespoons
  almond meal
16 tablespoons orris
  root
1 pint (570ml) milk

Whisk all the ingredients together for several minutes, until they are well blended. Pot up, label and refrigerate.

Add a cupful to the warm bath water. Soaking in this very luxurious milk gives one a gorgeously spoiled feeling, and transports one to the idyllic eastern surroundings where Cleopatra bathed in milk and almonds.

Honey and Oatmeal Beauty Bath Soak

1 tablespoon
  oatmeal
1 tablespoon honey

Mix the two ingredients together in a heavy mug or pan. Place the container and its contents underneath the warm water tap, and as you run a warm bath allow the tap water to run into the receptacle and brim over into the bath. This will ensure that the soak is completely dissolved, and evenly distributed. Remove the empty container, slide down into the silky mixture, put your head back, and relax for fifteen minutes.

This heavenly soak leaves the skin feeling like satin, and calms, soothes, and relaxes the most highly strung nerves. It encourages deep, peaceful sleep, too.

Mustard Tonic Bath Mix

Place the flowers in a saucepan, and pour the boiling water over them. Cover, and simmer for thirty minutes. Remove from the heat, and leave to steep for one hour. Strain, and stir the mustard powder into the liquid. Keep agitating until the powder has dissolved, then pour a pint (570ml) into the bath water, lie back, and immerse yourself for fifteen minutes.

8 flat tablespoons mustard powder
8 tablespoons dried camomile flowers
2 pints (1.15 litres) boiling water

Not only is this bath a wonderful tonic, but it is particularly beneficial for those who feel that they have the first symptoms of a cold or chill. In such cases, the best time to indulge yourself, is last thing at night, just prior to retiring.

Below I list many more enjoyable bath infusions. To make these, simply infuse a handful of the leaves or flowers in three pints of boiling water.

Infusion	Effect
Blackberry leaves	tones and invigorates
Camomile	relaxes and cleanses
Elderflowers	refreshes and cleanses
Horsetail	heals
Houseleek	heals and nourishes
Hyssop	pleasant-smelling tonic
Lavender flowers	pleasant-smelling tonic
Lemon verbena	pleasant-smelling tonic
Lovage	refreshes and is good for skin disorders
Rosemary	stimulates
Sweet basil	pleasant-smelling tonic
Valerian	helps cure insomnia
Yarrow	heals

Natural ingredients suitable for use in bath bags include the following:

Substance	Effect
Almond meal	heals and moisturizes
Barley	soothes and heals
Bicarbonate of soda	deep-cleanses
Bran	softens
Cornmeal	softens. Gentle to the most sensitive skins
Corn starch	relaxes
Dried milk	softens and nourishes
Epsom salts	deep-cleanses and relieves fatigue. Good for rheumatism
Honey	softens and relieves fatigue
Kitchen salt	softens, cleanses and relieves fatigue
Oatmeal	softens, cleanses and tones
Tea	soothes and heals

Many oils can be used individually as bath oils. These include:

almond oil
avocado oil
castor oil (treated)
castor oil (untreated)
cod liver oil
glycerine

linseed oil
olive oil
safflower oil
sesame oil
sunflower oil
turkey red oil

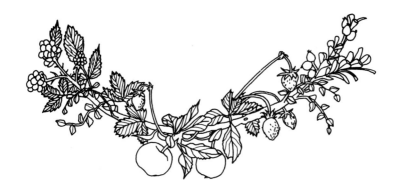

GELS AND SOAP SUBSTITUTES

The basis of all the gels and soaps in this section is ordinary manufactured soap, which I have added to and enriched with pure, natural ingredients.

My reasons for not providing a single, complete soap-making recipe are quite simple. No true soap, however pure, can be produced without one essential ingredient, caustic soda. This powdery substance is an alkali that unfortunately is an extremely strong skin irritant unless diluted. To obtain good or safe results when using it to make soap, it must be measured very carefully and treated with great respect. Any splashed on the skin can cause a nasty burn if not immediately washed away with vinegar or water. For this reason alone, I feel that the majority of people would be reluctant to handle this substance, especially since soap substitutes and gels such as mine are so much more gentle and kind to the skin. The additional natural ingredients they include greatly reduce any harmful or drying effects that the original soaps may have.

These soap substitutes are easy to make and they feel gorgeous on the skin. Many of you will wish to add your own favourite perfumed oils just prior to bottling or moulding, but often these 'soaps' have irresistible perfumes of their own — those containing honey are amongst my favourites — so I have rarely included any specific aromatic oils. Whether you do or don't depends entirely on you.

Honey and Olive Oil Soap Substitute

Place the soap in a double boiler or similar container on a low heat. Stir the soap with a wooden spoon. When melted, add the olive oil a few drops at a time. Once well blended, add the clear honey. Keep stirring the bubbling mixture for several minutes until it thickens, and then remove from the heat. Pour the liquid into a suitable mould and leave it to stand. When it has become hard — and this can take up to several weeks — it is ready for use.

9 tablespoons shredded castile soap
¾ teaspoon olive oil
1½ teaspoons clear honey

I always make this soap with no perfume at all because I adore the way it imparts a sweet smell of honey to the skin. It is a miraculous moisturizer and if, when rinsing your body, the water simply rolls off like water off a duck's back, don't worry, for that is exactly how it should be. Just towel your body dry, and you skin will feel beautifully soft and silky.

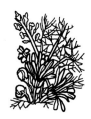

Oatmeal Powdered Soap with Lemon

2 tablespoons fine
oatmeal flakes
2 tablespoons kaolin
powder
½ teaspoonful borax
A few drops of oil of
lemon

Stir all the ingredients together. Pot up and label.

Sprinkle the powder on to either a loofah or face cloth, and using circular movements, massage it over your face as you would ordinary soap.

Sunflower Soap Substitute

8 tablespoons
shredded castile
soap
3 teaspoons
sunflower oil
3 teaspoons honey
A few drops of
sesame oil

Place the soap in a double boiler or similar container. Stir the soap with a wooden spoon until it has melted, and add the sunflower oil and honey. Continue stirring for a further seven to eight minutes, add the sesame oil, and remove from the heat. Pour the liquid into a suitable mould, and leave it in a warm room. It will be fit for use immediately it feels firm and hard. Alternatively, use it earlier as an ordinary soft soap.

Blackberry Bath Gel

1½ handfuls clean
blackberry leaves
6 tablespoons
shredded castile
soap
3 pints (1.7 litres)
soft water

Place the blackberry leaves in a pan, and pour the water over them. Bring the liquid to the boil, cover, and leave to simmer for ten minutes. Remove from the heat, and allow to steep for one-and-a-half to two hours. Strain. Return the blackberry infusion to the stove, and whilst it is bubbling, add the soap, and continue whisking all the time until the soap has become absorbed. When cool, bottle, label and refrigerate. Ready for use after two to three days.

I realize that blackberry leaves neither smell nor appear terribly exciting, but they are useful nevertheless, for those whose skins are prone to eruptions.

Lavender Bath Gel

Using a pestle or similar tool, crush the lavender heads until they are reduced to a powder. Put the soap and water in a pan or heat resistant bowl and, stirring frequently, leave to stand until they have blended. Stir in the powdered lavender and oil of lavender. Bottle and label. Smells gorgeous!

2½ tablespoons dried lavender heads
10 tablespoons finely shredded castile soap
8 tablespoons boiling water
4 drops oil of lavender

Herbal Bubble Bath Gel

Strain the herbal infusion into a pan, place on a low heat, and add the soap. Next, mix the glycerine, witch hazel, and eucalyptus oil together in a separate container. Once the soap in the mixture is thoroughly dissolved, combine the two liquids, remove from the heat, and whisk well. Beat in the gelatine, and when cool, pot up and label.

When running a bath, scoop a little of the bath gel into a heavy container and position it directly underneath the hot water bath tap. It will foam up into a gorgeous bubbly and fragrant froth and become dispersed into the bath.

¾ pint (425ml) herbal infusion containing angelica, comfrey, sweet cicely, and sweet woodruff
10 tablespoons shredded castile soap
3 tablespoons glycerine
4 teaspoons witch hazel
6 drops eucalyptus oil
2 tablespoons powdered gelatine

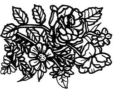

Liquid Mint Soap with Glycerine

Place the shredded soap and water together in a double boiler or similar container and bring to the boil. When the soap has completely dissolved, stir in the glycerine. Remove from the heat and blend in the mint oil. When cool, pot and label.

8 tablespoons castile soap, shredded
1 pint (570ml) soft water
5 tablespoons glycerine
4 drops mint oil

Soapwort Bath Shampoo with Herbs

4 tablespoons soapwort root, crushed
4 tablespoons mixed herbs
2 pints (1.15 litres) boiling water

Place the soapwort and other herbs together in a heat-resistant bowl and add the boiling water. Cover and leave for thirty minutes. Strain, bottle and label.

To use, pour out the soap liquid and wash in the usual way.

Soapwort is one of the purest and most natural cleansers. This basic recipe may be used to produce many other body and hair shampoos, as long as you have ample soapwort root at your disposal.

Pine Bath Gel

1½ handfuls pine cones, crushed
3 pints (1.7 litres) soft water
6 tablespoons castile soap, shredded

Place the cones in a saucepan and pour the water over them. Bring to the boil, cover, and simmer for ten minutes. Remove from the heat and allow to infuse for two hours. Strain. Boil the pine infusion again, add the soap and continue whisking until all traces of the soap have disappeared. When cool, pot, label and refrigerate. Leave for a few days and then use as a soft soap.

Eucalyptus Bath Gel

1½ handfuls clean eucalyptus leaves
3 pints (1.7 litres) soft water
6 tablespoons castile soap, shredded

Place the eucalyptus leaves in a pot and pour the water over them. Bring to the boil, cover and simmer for about ten to fifteen minutes. Remove from the heat and infuse for one and a half to two hours. Strain. Boil the infusion again and while the liquid is bubbling, add the soap. Whisk all the time until all soap has dissolved. When cool, pot, label and refrigerate. Use as a soft soap.

This delightfully fragrant gel helps to soothe tired muscles and reduce fatigue.

Almond Bath Gel

2½ tablespoons almonds
10 tablespoons castile soap, finely shredded
8 tablespoons boiling water
4 drops almond oil

Crush the almonds with a pestle or similar tool until they are reduced to a fairly fine powder. Then place the soap and boiling water in a saucepan or heat-resistant bowl, stirring frequently until the soap has dissolved. Stir in the powdered almonds and oil of almonds. Pot and label. Use as a soft soap.

BODY OILS AND LOTIONS

Apricot Body Oil with Cinnamon

Pour the ingredients into a jar, cork firmly and shake until the oils have merged. Label.

    This wonderfully aromatic oil may be applied to any dry areas of the body, but it is really too luxurious to use solely as a body moisturizer! I indulge myself by spreading a fine film of it over my face and neck, concentrating on any tell-tale lines and wrinkles. Within a few hours, any such imperfections have usually disappeared.

8 tablespoons apricot oil
3 drops cinnamon oil

Orangeflower Body Lotion

Place the borax in the rosewater, stir until all powdery traces have disappeared, and then blend in the warm oil. Whisk continuously for several minutes until the lotion is well mixed. Only then stir in the orangeflower water. Bottle and label.

1 teaspoon borax
½ pint (285ml) rosewater
2 tablespoons warm olive oil
4–5 teaspoons orangeflower water

Rosewater and Glycerine Body Lotion

Beat the ingredients together until the lotion is well mixed. Bottle and label.

    Rosewater and glycerine together make a super all-over body moisturizer. This lotion has been used for centuries to soften and nourish the skin, and particularly the face, neck, and hands.

6 tablespoons rosewater
2 tablespoons glycerine

Sesame Body Oil

Mix the ingredients, bottle and label. Put the bottle in an obvious place to remind you to shake the contents well several times a day. This will release the woody aroma of the benzoin.

8 tablespoons sesame oil
2 tablespoons powdered gum benzoin

Castor and Coconut Body Oil

4 tablespoons
  coconut oil
1 tablespoon almond
  oil
2 tablespoons castor
  oil
Perfumed oil
  (optional)

Melt the coconut oil in a double saucepan and stir. When runny, remove from the heat and beat in the almond and castor oils. Continue beating until the individual liquid is homogenous. If you like, stir in the perfumed oil of your choice. Bottle and label.

Lanolin and Almond Body Oil

8 tablespoons
  lanolin
4 tablespoons
  almond oil
Perfumed oil
  (optional)

Melt the lanolin over a low heat and then stir in the almond oil. Whisk. When cool beat in a few drops of the perfumed oil of your choice. Bottle and label.

After-Bath Body Oil

12 teaspoons
  sunflower oil
8 teaspoons
  safflower oil
8 teaspoons almond
  oil
4 teaspoons maize
  oil
4 teaspoons olive oil
Perfumed oil as
  required

Whip well together. Bottle and label.

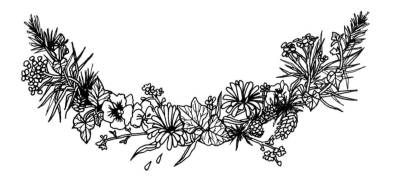

I have given recipes for only a few simple body oils and lotions because both the day and night moisturizing face creams and the lighter nourishing skin milks described also make excellent body creams and lotions.

Other natural products that may be massaged into the body include:

almond oil	lanolin	safflower oil
avocado oil	maize oil	soya oil
cocoa butter (melted)	milk	sunflower oil
coconut oil	olive oil	vegetable margarine
corn oil	peach oil	(melted)
dairy cream	peanut oil	wheatgerm oil
glycerine	rosewater	

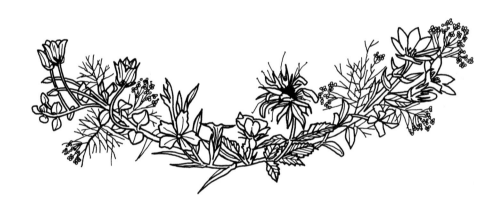

13

For Sunbathing

SUNTAN OILS

Deep Suntan Oil

3 tablespoons
coconut oil
3 tablespoons cocoa
butter
6 tablespoons sesame
oil
3 tablespoons olive
oil
2 tablespoons
almond oil
1 pint (570ml) extra
strong cold Indian
tea

Place the coconut oil and the cocoa butter together in a double boiler and melt over a low heat. Pour in the remaining oils and blend. Remove from the heat and pour in the tea. Whisk the mixture for several minutes. Bottle and label. Always shake well before use.

French Suntan Oil

8 tablespoons
coconut oil
8 drops bergamot oil

Melt the coconut oil in a double boiler. Remove from the heat and stir in the bergamot oil. Whip until cool. Bottle and label.

This is a favourite oil amongst the sun-worshipping French. It smells expensive and wildly exotic!

Inexpensive Suntan Lotion with Iodine

Place the oils, vinegar, and iodine into an electric blender or mixing bowl and whisk for several minutes. Add the sweet-smelling jasmine or alternative aromatic oil. Blend, bottle and label.

8 tablespoons sesame oil
4 tablespoons corn oil
4 tablespoons sunflower oil
8 tablespoons cider vinegar
1 teaspoon iodine
A few drops jasmine oil or some similar fragrance

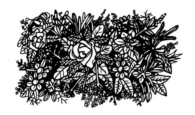

Lavender Suntan Oil

Pour all the ingredients into either an ordinary mixing bowl, or an electric blender if you have one, and whisk furiously for several minutes. Bottle and label.

The lavender oil not only imparts a gorgeous aroma, but also discourages flying mites such as hungry midges and bloodthirsty mosquitoes from landing and feasting on our tender torsos!

6 tablespoons sesame oil
4 tablespoons olive oil
2 tablespoons cider vinegar
A few drops lavender oil

A Fine Tanning Oil with Lanolin

Place the lanolin in a double boiler or similar container, over a low heat, and when it has melted, stir in the oil and water simultaneously. For this operation, it is best if a friend or a member of the family whisks the ingredients, which will give you two free hands for the oil and water. Continue stirring for a minute or two until the mixture is thoroughly blended. Bottle, label and refrigerate. Always shake well before use.

8 tablespoons sesame oil
8 tablespoons anhydrous lanolin
¾ pint (425ml) water

Coconut Suntan Oil

Place the oil and cocoa butter together in a double boiler and melt over a low heat. Remove from the heat and blend in the lavender oil. Whisk until cool. Bottle and label.

6 tablespoons coconut oil
6 tablespoons cocoa butter
A few drops lavender oil

Tea Tanning Oil

6 tablespoons sesame
oil or tahini
2½ tablespoons
coconut oil
2½ tablespoons
lanolin
8 tablespoons very
strong, cold
Indian tea

Place the oils and the lanolin in a double boiler or similar container and gently heat them until they have melted and mixed together. Remove from the heat and pour in the cold tea. Whisk well, bottle and label. Shake well before use.

The natural dye in tea encourages the skin to tan more quickly. The most important of the ingredients, however, is sesame oil, which contains a natural screening agent which absorbs harmful ultra-violet rays, thereby preventing sunburn. The above quantities will produce well over half a pint (300ml), and although the recipe is no miracle-worker, it will be invaluable for any suntanning session.

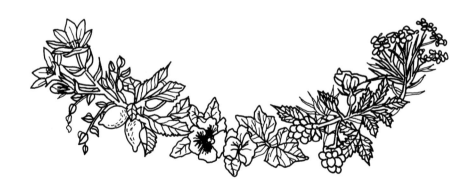

174

SUNBURN LOTIONS

Honey Heat Lotion

Mix all the ingredients together and apply to areas of sunburn.

1 egg white
1 teaspoon clear,
runny honey
½ teaspoon witch
hazel

Olive Oil Lotion with Eucalyptus Oil

Whip the olive oil and glycerine together. When blended, add the eucalyptus oil. Apply directly to sunburned skin.

1 tablespoon olive
oil
1 tablespoon
glycerine
2 drops eucalyptus
oil

Strawberry Sunburn Splash

Using a fork, mash the strawberries and apply the pulp liberally over the sunburned face or body until the affected areas feel quite wet. Leave the treated areas for thirty minutes. Then splash with a soothing solution of tepid water and tincture of benzoin. Pat dry.

Squashed strawberries also make a marvellous natural dentifrice. Any soft ones left over at any time should be brushed on to the teeth. They remove plaque and stains and will return teeth to their original pearly whiteness.

2 large juicy
strawberries
A few drops tincture
of benzoin
Lukewarm water

Calamine and Glycerine Sunburn Lotion

Whisk the ingredients together thoroughly. Bottle and label. Shake well before each application.

12½ tablespoons
water
10 teaspoons
calamine
2½ teaspoons
glycerine

Quince Sunburn Gel

4 tablespoons water
2 tablespoons quince seeds

Place the seeds in a bowl, and pour the water over them. Leave to steep, stirring occasionally, until a jelly-like substance forms. Strain, and apply the healing, soothing gel to the affected areas.

This substance also softens the skin, and any unused residue should be compounded in your favourite night or day cream.

Other soothing sunburn remedies include:

    witch hazel compress
    apple cider vinegar compress
    raw potato juice compress
    cold tea compress
    sage tea compress
    cucumber juice compress
    white wine compress
    buttermilk compress
    gin compress
    cornflour (sprinkle powder over affected areas)

There are also several soothing infusions (in each case use one tablespoonful to eight tablespoons boiling water):

    lettuce leaves
    nettle leaves
    elderflower leaves and/or berries
    camomile flowers
    cowslip flowers

A dilution of one tablespoon vinegar to eight tablespoons water is also effective.

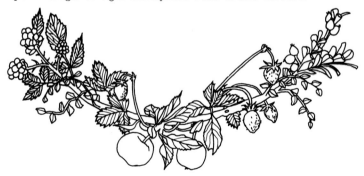

14
Colognes and Floral Water

Some people find great pleasure in brewing and sampling home-made wines and over the years I, too, have experimented with alcoholic brews and produced a small but good selection of sweet-smelling colognes and floral waters. Like wines, they may be sampled at any time after reaching maturity and on occasion used lavishly. They are far less expensive, and more individual, than many of their manufactured equivalents. Always use a pipette for measuring oils.

In a fairly short time you can build up a delightful collection of fragrances to suit your every mood. Once you have made the initial outlay on aromatic oils and alcohol, you'll discover that this rewarding hobby is nothing like as costly as you imagine.

Eau de Lavender

Pour the lavender oil and rosewater into the alcohol. Shake well, bottle and label. Store in a cool, dark place and shake the bottle daily. It may be used after a month, but the more time it is given to mature the better.

1 teaspoon lavender oil
6 tablespoons rosewater
½ pint (285ml) alcohol

Lavender and Bergamot Cologne

¾ tablespoon
  ambergris essence
1 tablespoon
  bergamot essence
1 tablespoon
  lavender oil
1 pint (570ml) wine
  spirit

Pour the essences and oil into the spirit. Shake well, bottle and label. Store in a cool, dark place, and remember to shake daily. This cologne may be used after three months but, like wine, it improves with age.

Mint and Rosemary Cologne

2 tablespoons fresh
  mint
2 tablespoons fresh
  rosemary
Peel of ½ lemon,
  grated
Peel of ½ orange,
  grated
8 tablespoons
  alcohol
½ pint (285ml)
  rosewater

Place all the ingredients together in a bottle, cork and leave to steep for ten days. Strain, rebottle and label. It may be used immediately the ten days have elapsed, but don't forget to shake daily during that period.

Eau de Bergamot

2 teaspoons
  bergamot oil
1¼ teaspoons sweet
  orange oil
2½ teaspoons orris
7 drops rosemary oil
1½ teaspoons lemon
  oil
1¼ teaspoons
  benzoin
50 drops neroli oil
2½ pints (1.4 litres)
  alcohol

Place all the ingredients together in an airtight container and let them macerate for six months. Shake the container every day. After this time has elapsed, strain, bottle and label. Store in a cool dark place. It may be used immediately.

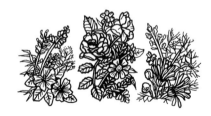

Eau de Ylang-Ylang

Pour all the ingredients into a bottle, cork well and store in a cool, dark place. Shake the contents daily for four months. Then strain, rebottle and label. Leave for a further three months before use.

20 drops ylang-ylang essence
10 drops rose geranium oil
10 drops patchouli oil
1 pint (570ml) alcohol

Eau de Spices

Pour the oils into the alcohol. Shake well, bottle and label. Store in a cool, dark place, and make sure you shake the cologne daily.

The preparation may be used after four months, but the longer you keep it the more mature it becomes.

10 drops cinnamon oil
10 drops clove oil
½ pint (285ml) alcohol

Bergamot and Clove Cologne

Pour the oils into the alcohol. Shake well, bottle and label. Store in a cool, dark place and don't forget the daily shake.

This delightful herb-smelling cologne improves with age. If you are in a rush, you may sample it after four months, but try to keep it longer if you can — it will be well worth the wait.

20 drops bergamot oil
20 drops clove oil
1 pint (570ml) alcohol

Sweet Orange Cologne

Pour all the ingredients into an airtight container and store in a cool, dark place for six months. Shake the container every day. After this long wait has elapsed, strain, bottle and label. Leave for several more months before use.

½ pint (285ml) alcohol
1½ teaspoons bergamot oil
½ teaspoon benzoin
5 teaspoons sweet orange oil
¾ teaspoon lemon oil
15 drops rose geranium oil

Zingy Spice Water

2 pints (1.15 litres)
white wine
vinegar
16 tablespoons
crushed cloves
2 pints (1.15 litres)
rosewater
6 bay leaves,
crushed

Pour all the ingredients into a saucepan, cover and bring to the boil. Leave to simmer for one hour. During this time check the liquid level every ten minutes or so, and replace that lost through evaporation with plain water. After simmering remove the pan from the heat, allow to cool, bottle and label. Store in a cool, dark place and agitate the bottle every day for three months.

The liquid may then be strained and rebottled. Leave for a further few months — the longer the better — before using it.

Floral Water with Verbena

2 pints (1.15 litres)
alcohol
¼ pint (140ml)
orange flower
water
30 drops rosemary
oil
15 drops lime oil
¼ pint rosewater
1¾ teaspoons
verbena oil
23 drops orange oil
7 drops peppermint
oil

Pour all the ingredients into an airtight container and store in a cool and dark place for six months. Shake the contents daily — it's a bore, but it's important — and once the necessary time has elapsed, strain, bottle and label. Leave for a further two to three months before use.

Eau d'Orange

12 drops orange oil
8 drops bergamot oil
4 drops lavender oil
4 drops ambergris
tincture
1 pint (570ml)
alcohol

Pour the oils and tincture into the alcohol. Shake well, bottle and label. Store in a cool dark place, remembering to give the contents a daily shake.

It may be used after four months, but it will continue to improve if given six more! Indeed, the longer it is kept, the richer it becomes.

Lemon Balm Water

Mix the leaves, peel, allspice and alcohol together in an airtight container. Secure the lid tightly, and leave it to steep for ten days. Then strain and add the water. Bottle, shake well and label. May be used immediately.

This is an invigorating and refreshing balm water, so always try to keep a small bottle of it in your handbag.

8 tablespoons crushed lemon balm leaves
4 tablespoons finely shredded lemon peel
½ teaspoon allspice
½ pint (285ml) alcohol
¾ pint (425ml) soft water

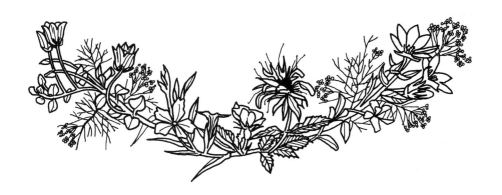

181

15

For the Feet

Deodorizing Herbal Foot Bath

2 tablespoons
rosemary
2 tablespoons
pennyroyal
2 tablespoons sage
2 tablespoons
angelica
2 tablespoons
juniper berries
2 pints (1.15 litres)
boiling water

Put all the ingredients in the boiling water, cover and leave to stand for one hour. Strain, bottle and refrigerate.

Pour half a pint (285ml) of liquid into a foot-basin partially filled with warm water. Immerse your feet in the soak for fifteen to twenty minutes. Pat dry and apply a cologne or astringent.

Lady's Bedstraw Foot Bath

1 handful lady's
bedstraw
1 pint (570ml)
boiling water

Soak the lady's bedstraw in the water for ten minutes. Strain, bottle and refrigerate.

Pour half a pint (285ml) of liquid into a foot-bath partially filled with warm water. Immerse your feet in the soak, and leave them until all the tiredness has been drawn away. Pat dry and apply a little alcohol or rosemary oil to your feet.

Mixed Herbal Foot Mix for Aching Feet

Mix all the herbs together and pot in an airtight jar. When your feet ache badly, take three tablespoonsful of this herbal mixture and pour it into four pints (2.3 litres) of boiling water. Cover and simmer over a low heat for five minutes. Remove from the heat and allow to stew for twenty minutes. Strain, and pour the infusion into a foot-bath.

When the liquid has cooled sufficiently, immerse your feet in it. They will soon feel relieved. Pat dry and apply a suitable soothing treatment such as marigold oil.

5 tablespoons dried marjoram
7 tablespoons dried peppermint
3 tablespoons dried thyme
5 tablespoons dried camomile
4 tablespoons dried rosemary

Foot Oil for Aching Feet

Mix the oils together, bottle and label. Massage well into the feet.

5 tablespoons sesame oil
6 drops clove oil

Several herbs can be infused to make effective soaks for tired and aching feet. In each case infuse one handful in two pints (1.15 litres) of boiling water.

Infusion	Use
Elderberry leaves	Add half pint (285ml) of this liquid to the foot-bath water.
Horsetail	Add half pint (285ml) of this liquid to the foot-bath water together with 1 tablespoon sea salt.
Lavender leaves	Add half pint (285ml) of this liquid to the foot-bath water.
Lime (linden)flowers	Add half pint (285ml) of this liquid to the foot-bath water.
Nettles	Add half pint (285ml) of this liquid to the foot-bath water.
Marigold leaves	Add half pint (285ml) of this liquid to the foot-bath water.
Others include:	
Cider vinegar	Add quarter pint (140ml) to the foot-bath water.
Epsom salts and borax	Add 2 tablespoon epsom salts and 1 tablespoon borax to the foot-bath water.
Mustard	Add 2 teaspoonful to the foot-bath water.
Sea salt	Add 2 tablespoonsful to the foot-bath water.
Washing soda and dried lavender	Add 1 tablespoon soda and 4 tablespoons lavender to the foot-bath water.

Infusions of blackberry or oak leaves make deodorizing foot-bath soaks. In each case infuse one handful in 2 pints (1.15 litres) boiling water. Pour half a pint (285ml) of the liquid into the foot-bath water.

ABC Of Herbs and Plants and Their Growing Requirements

Popular name	Latin name	Type of plant	Planting/ sowing season	Garden soil	Alternative growing mixture	Position	Propagation
Angelica	Angelica archangelica	Biennial/ perennial	September & April	Deep moist loam	JIP or Lev. No. 2	Shade	By seed or offsets
Basil (sweet)	Ocimum basilicum	Annual	March/April	Light, well-drained soil	JIP or Lev. No. 2	Sunny sheltered position	By seed
Bay	Laurus nobilis	Evergreen shrub	March/April	Rich, porous loam	JIP or Lev. No. 2 or 3	Sunny sheltered position	By heel cuttings
Carrot	Daucus carota	Annual	March-July	Deep, light rich soil	Equal parts by volume of rich loam, well-rotted manure and leafmould	Sun or partial shade	By seed
Cucumber	Cucumis sativus	Annual	Varies according to the strain	Rich, moist open soil	2 parts loam and 1 part stable manure	Partial shade	By seed
Eucalyptus	Eucalyptus globulus	Evergreen shrub/tree	June/July	Well-drained fertile soil	JIP or Lev. No.3	Full sun	By seed
Fennel	Foeniculum vulgare	Perennial	March, April & May	Fertile, well-drained soil	JIP or Lev. No. 2	Full sun	By seed or division
Houseleek	Sempervivum tectorum	Evergreen succulent	September/ October and March/April	Well-drained soil	Equal parts of JIP or Lev. No. 2 and coarse sand	Full sun	By offsets or seed
Lavender	Lavendula spica	Evergreen shrub	September-March	Well-drained soil	JIP or Lev. No. 2 or 3	Full sun	By seed or stem cutting
Lettuce	Lactuca sativa	Annual	Varies according to the strain	Fertile, well-drained soil	JIP or Lev. No. 2 or 3	Sun or shade	By seed

Popular name	Latin name	Type of plant	Planting/ sowing season	Garden soil	Alternative growing mixture	Position	Propagation
Marigold	Calendula officinalis	Annual	March or September	Well-drained soil	JIP or Lev. No. 2	Sun	By seed
Mint	Mentha spp.	Perennial	October- March	Rich, moist soil	JIP or Lev. No. 2 or 3	Sun or partial shade	By division
Parsley	Carum petroselinum crispum	Biennial	February- August	Well-drained fertile soil	JIP or Lev. No. 2 or 3	Sun or partial shade	By seed
Potato	Solanum tuberosum	Perennial	April onwards	Rich, moist soil	JIP or Lev. No. 3	Sun or partial shade	By tubers
Rhubarb	Rheum rhaponticum or R. officinale	Perennial	March	Ordinary soil	JIP or Lev. No. 2 or 3	Sun or partial shade	By seed or division
Rose	Rosa	Varies according to the strain					
Rosemary	Rosmarinus officinalis	Evergreen shrub	September or March	Light, dry soil	JIP or Lev. No. 2	Full sun	By cuttings of mature growth
Sage	Salvia officinalis	Evergreen sub-shrub	March and April	Well-drained light soil	JIP or Lev. No. 2 or 3	Full sun	By heel cuttings or seed
Southernwood	Artemisia abrotanum	Deciduous or semi-evergreen shrub	March and April	Well-drained fertile soil	JIP or Lev. No. 2 or 3	Sun	By semi-hard wood heel cuttings
Strawberry	Fragaria × ananassa	Perennial	June and July	Rich soil	JIP or Lev. No. 2 or 3	Full sun	By runners
Sweet Cicely	Myrrhis odorata	Perennial	March/April	Well-drained soil	JIP or Lev. No. 2	Partial shade	By seed or division
Thyme	Thymus vulgaris	Evergreen perennial	March/April	Well-drained soil	JIP or Lev. No. 1 or 2	Full sun	By division, heel cuttings, layering or seed
Tomato	Lycopersicon esculentum	Annual	March/April	Rich, moist soil	JIP or Lev. No. 3	Sunny, sheltered spot	By seed

Note: Lev. = Levingtons

Equipment for Making Your Own Cosmetics

You can see from the list below that most of the equipment needed for making cosmetics will probably be found in your kitchen.

Equipment	Use
Enamel double boiler *or* a heat-resistant glass bowl which will fit into an enamel saucepan	For melting waxes and oils over a very low heat. Never use aluminium pans
Several heat-resistant bowls of differing sizes	As above
Wooden spoon, tablespoon, dessertspoon, teaspoon, fork and potato masher	Mixing and measuring
Electric blender *or* egg whisk	Thorough mixing and blending
Pestle and mortar *or* bowl and crushing tool such as a spoon	Crushing and grinding
Liquidizer	Making your own pure fruit and vegetable juices can save you a lot of money, and this should be considered an investment
An ample supply of clean jars, tubs and bottles of varying sizes	To store all your creams and lotions
Eye dropper	For adding aromatic oils
Good pouring jug and small funnel	To ensure that you don't spill any liquids when bottling them
Plastic scraper	Necessary for scooping out the last traces of creams into the jars

Equipment	Use
Kitchen grater	For grating beeswax, etc.
Fine sieve *or* some muslin	For straining infusions
Self-adhesive sticky labels	Be sure to label each jar as soon as you use it
Moulds	Only necessary if you intend to make hard soaps and lip salves

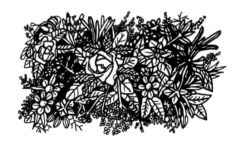

Index

188

189

191